Managing Concussions in Schools

Susan C. Davies, EdD, NCSP, is an Associate Professor and Coordinator of the School Psychology Program at the University of Dayton, Dayton, Ohio. A nationally certified school psychologist, she is the founder and coordinator of the National Association of School Psychologists (NASP) Traumatic Brain Injury Interest Group. Dr. Davies currently advises the Ohio Department of Health on developing and leading a return-to-learn concussion team model for Ohio schools. She also served as a participant in the Centers for Disease Control and Prevention's Expert Concussion Workgroup and as a reviewer of the American Academy of Neurology's revised sport concussion policy. She has over 15 years of experience in the field of school psychology as a practicing psychologist, program evaluator, and university faculty member. The primary focus of her research addresses traumatic brain injuries (TBIs) in school populations, including such issues as increasing educator awareness of TBI, efficacy of specific interventions, and developing model service plans for students with TBI. Her work has been published in such peer-reviewed publications as *Journal of Educational and Psychological Consultation, Contemporary School Psychology, Physical Disabilities and Related Services, School Psychology Forum, Psychology in the Schools, Journal of Applied School Psychology, Brain Injury,* and *Best Practices in School Psychology: Systems-Level Services*, the flagship manual of the profession. She is the coauthor (with Paul Jantz and Erin Bigler) of *Working with Traumatic Brain Injury in Schools* (2014). She has presented on this topic at national and regional conferences as well as providing in-service training to educators.

Managing Concussions in Schools

A Guide to Recognition, Response, and Leadership

SUSAN C. DAVIES, EdD, NCSP

SPRINGER PUBLISHING COMPANY
NEW YORK

Copyright © 2016 Springer Publishing Company, LLC

All rights reserved.

No part of this publication may be reproduced, stored in a retrieval system, or transmitted in any form or by any means, electronic, mechanical, photocopying, recording, or otherwise, without the prior permission of Springer Publishing Company, LLC, or authorization through payment of the appropriate fees to the Copyright Clearance Center, Inc., 222 Rosewood Drive, Danvers, MA 01923, 978-750-8400, fax 978-646-8600, info@copyright.com or on the Web at www.copyright.com.

Springer Publishing Company, LLC
11 West 42nd Street
New York, NY 10036
www.springerpub.com

Acquisitions Editor: Nancy Hale
Composition: diacriTech

ISBN: 978-0-8261-6922-8
e-book ISBN: 978-0-8261-6923-5

Student Supplements are available from springerpub.com/Davies
Forms and Handouts: 978-0-8261-6924-2

16 17 18 19 20 / 5 4 3 2 1

The author and the publisher of this Work have made every effort to use sources believed to be reliable to provide information that is accurate and compatible with the standards generally accepted at the time of publication. The author and publisher shall not be liable for any special, consequential, or exemplary damages resulting, in whole or in part, from the readers' use of, or reliance on, the information contained in this book. The publisher has no responsibility for the persistence or accuracy of URLs for external or third-party Internet websites referred to in this publication and does not guarantee that any content on such websites is, or will remain, accurate or appropriate.

Library of Congress Cataloging-in-Publication Data

Names: Davies, Susan C., author.
Title: Managing concussions in schools : a front-line guide to recognition, response, and leadership / Susan C. Davies.
Description: New York, NY : Springer Publishing Company, LLC, [2016] | Includes bibliographical references and index.
Identifiers: LCCN 2016013690 | ISBN 9780826169228 | ISBN 9780826169235 (e-ISBN)
Subjects: | MESH: Brain Concussion—prevention & control | School Health Services
Classification: LCC RC394.C7 | NLM WL 354 | DDC 617.4/81044—dc23 LC record available at http://lccn.loc.gov/2016013690

Special discounts on bulk quantities of our books are available to corporations, professional associations, pharmaceutical companies, health care organizations, and other qualifying groups. If you are interested in a custom book, including chapters from more than one of our titles, we can provide that service as well.
For details, please contact:
Special Sales Department, Springer Publishing Company, LLC
11 West 42nd Street, 15th Floor, New York, NY 10036-8002
Phone: 877-687-7476 or 212-431-4370; Fax: 212-941-7842
E-mail: sales@springerpub.com

Printed in the United States of America by McNaughton & Gunn.

CONTENTS

Preface *vii*

Acknowledgments *xi*

1. Overview of Concussions — 1
2. The Aftermath: Effects of Concussions — 21
3. The Concussion Team Model — 40
4. Concussion Assessment — 66
5. Recovery: Return to Academics, Return to Play — 94
6. Adjustments to the School Environment — 111
7. Prevention and Training — 137

Index *152*

PREFACE

Early one morning, I received a frantic call from my friend Beth.

"Joey got hit in the head really hard with a soccer ball during his game last night. He seemed okay at first and went back in to finish the half. But then he looked kind of queasy after the game was over—he didn't even want the snack afterward! And he was very quiet on the way home. He said he was fine, but then he went right to sleep. This morning he has a bad headache and he just wants to stay in bed. Do you think he has a concussion? Should I take him to the hospital?"

Beth was a coach, a parent, and a high school teacher. She had no idea what to do.

This was several years ago. Because of the prominence and number of news stories related to the potential dangers of concussions, laws have been passed in all states that require a return-to-play protocol for student athletes. As a coach, Beth is now required to attend concussion training; as a parent, she is required to sign a document verifying that she has read about concussions and understands the risk associated with her children's selected sports. As an educator, however, nothing definite is required of her. Like most teachers, Beth has received no specific training or professional development on what to do for classroom-related concerns if one of her students is suffering from the effects of a concussion.

The need for this book

There is an overall lack of understanding about concussions in school communities, as well as a lack of understanding about how to support a student with a known concussion. Despite widespread media attention and increased scientific scrutiny, concussions remain a source of misunderstanding and controversy. While a number of reputable online resources provide guidance to help students return to school postconcussion (see Chapter 7), there was a need for a single comprehensive text to provide guidance to school-based professionals as they navigate the barriers, system issues, knowledge gaps, and complexities in recognizing and responding to student concussions. And while there were a number of existing books that addressed traumatic brain injuries (TBIs) broadly, none focused exclusively on helping school-based professionals recognize and respond to concussion.

Because there is no bandage or cast, it can be difficult for educators to fully understand the needs of the student with a concussion. *Just as we wouldn't expect a student who has broken a leg to run laps in gym class, we cannot expect the student with an injured brain to complete all of the mental exercises expected in a typical school day.* Students who have sustained concussions typically need a short-term plan upon their return to school that meets both their academic and physical needs. This is different from the approach we take for students with moderate or severe TBIs. In those cases, the transition may take place over a much longer period of time and require more intensive modifications to the curriculum.

All adults in the school community—everyone from teachers to school psychologists, from coaches to bus drivers, and from administrators to school nurses—need to better understand the signs and symptoms of concussion so they can respond effectively when a student is injured at school. Additionally, educators often encounter situations involving students who sustained a concussion off of school grounds, but who return to school while symptomatic. Although this book was primarily written for school psychologists, counselors, administrators, and nurses, it can also serve as a valuable resource for teachers, athletic staff, parents, students, and any other key participants in a successful recovery process. In addition to serving as an indispensable resource for school teams, this book can also serve as a supplemental book for graduate-level training programs in school leadership, school psychology, and school counseling, as well as for nursing programs that prepare school-based practitioners.

Overview

The *primary objectives* of this book are to provide school personnel with the following:

- Information on how concussions can affect learning, mental health, and social–emotional functioning
- Skills in developing and leading a school-based concussion support team
- Tools for school-based concussion assessment
- Information on a safe, gradual process of returning to the academic environment

- Guidelines for creating symptom-based adjustments to the learning environment in collaboration with the family, community, and school team
- Resources for prevention and training initiatives

This book opens with a chapter that provides an overview of concussion: what happens to the brain at the moment of impact, terminology, prevalence rates, causes, risk factors, and issues related to underreporting of concussions. Chapter 1 also provides a section that dispells concussion myths and misconceptions. Chapter 2 reviews the effects of concussions, including invisible neurological changes and overt signs and symptoms. Educators will learn about developmental effects—how concussions can affect students of different ages—as well as persistent and severe difficulties that can result from concussions. Chapter 3 presents a school-based concussion team model, including the structure of the team and the specific roles and responsibilities of each team member—particularly the concussion team leader. Chapter 4 describes concussion assessment tools. Readers will become familiar with checklists that can be used within the school, as well as testing that may occur in a medical facility, clinic, or at the sidelines of a sporting event. This chapter also describes assessment tools that can be used at the school for ongoing assessment and progress monitoring. Chapter 5 provides an overview of the concussion recovery process from the first days postinjury through return to school and play. Readers will learn about how physical and cognitive rest can be balanced with a return to activity. In Chapter 6, readers will learn about adjustments to the school environment that can benefit students who return to school while they are still symptomatic. It gives concussion team members guidance on the selection of appropriate strategies, as well as decision making during a student's return to academics. Finally, Chapter 7 is devoted to concussion prevention information. This chapter also provides guidance on how readers might train others on concussion recognition and response. Case studies are integrated throughout the chapters: Readers will follow the same four students from the point of injury through recovery. A number of forms are provided throughout the book, such as a signs and symptoms checklist, a postconcussion care plan, a checklist of academic adjustments, and progress monitoring tools; **copies of these forms are available for download at springerpub.com/Davies.**

ACKNOWLEDGMENTS

My heartfelt thanks to the following people for their contributions and support in creating this book: the school children and staff who inspired my work on this topic; Nancy Hale, my editor at Springer, who was interested in my work; my friends and concussion experts Sara Timms and Brenda Eagan Brown, who assisted in reviewing this manuscript; and my colleagues in the Department of Counselor Education and Human Services at the University of Dayton, who offered support and encouragement. Within that department, special thanks to Elana Bernstein—everyone should be so lucky as to have a friend like Elana at work—and to school psychology graduate students Amanda Prater, who jumped right in to help with this book on her first day of graduate school, and Maria Tedesco, who assisted with references and images. Special thanks and love to my parents, Fred and Becky Davies, who instilled in us a love for books, education, and children: My daughters fall asleep among a pile of books because of you. Most of all, thanks to my husband, Allen, and our six children, my sources of deepest joy and inspiration.

CHAPTER 1

Overview of Concussions

A concussion is a type of mild traumatic brain injury (mTBI) that can result in a constellation of problematic symptoms. These include cognitive, physical, emotional, social, and behavioral symptoms, all of which can affect students' well-being and performance in school. Concussions have received a great deal of media attention in recent years—largely due to controversies in professional sports regarding the long-term effects of concussions sustained by athletes. However, school-age children are at particularly high risk for sustaining brain injuries. This age group is also at higher risk for prolonged recovery (Gilchrist, Thomas, Xu, McGuire, & Coronado, 2011). Yet, despite the fact that concussions are relatively common injuries, educators typically receive little or no instruction in concussion recognition and response.

While some think of concussions as injuries that primarily occur in athletes, a number of school-age children sustain concussions through accidents, falls, fights, abuse, and everyday play. A student may come to school on Monday morning describing a car crash she was in over the weekend. She may tell her teacher about going to the emergency department (ED). She may say that she is very tired and she may seem noticeably distracted. But the teacher may not know whether the student is suffering from the effects of a head injury or if she is simply tired from a long night in the ED. The teacher may think the student is distracted simply because the crash and hospital events frightened her. Likewise, a school administrator may have a boy come to the office after a fight and, seeing no blood or broken bones, be so focused on the disciplinary ramifications that he or she misses the fact that the student is confused and answering questions slowly—classic signs of concussion.

Adding to such ambiguity is the reality that because every child is different, every concussion is different. Some students may have an "obvious" concussion and receive prompt and thorough medical evaluations. But others may not be diagnosed for days. Some may miss school and then have persistent symptoms that affect academic functioning; others may recover quickly and need very few short-term adjustments to their school routines.

The positive news medically is that, with appropriate diagnosis and management, a full recovery is possible for most youth who sustain concussions. Thus, school personnel working at all grade levels need to better understand their potential roles and responsibilities in assisting students who have sustained concussions. The purpose of this book is to provide a concise manual to assist teachers and other school staff members to support the return of students with concussions to their academic and extracurricular activities.

WHAT IS A CONCUSSION?

A concussion is the result of a bump or blow to the head—or one to the body—that causes the head to move rapidly back and forth, as illustrated in Figure 1.1. While we typically recognize concussive hits to the head—the fall on a hard surface, the whack with a hockey stick, the collision with the dashboard during a car accident—concussions frequently occur with no contact to the head at all. A hard blow to the body—for example, during a football tackle—can shake the brain in the skull cavity so much that it can cause a concussion. These forces may be linear and direct, which tend to snap the head backward and then forward, or they may be rotational, which can be more damaging because they cause the brain to rotate and spin within the skull. These forces can cause the blood vessels and brain tissue to stretch and shear.

These jolts can change the way the brain normally works because they result in a disruption of neurochemistry. The forceful movement to the head results in an alteration of mental status, which manifests as confusion or disorientation. Brain function is temporarily disrupted. However, because concussions are largely a neurometabolic injury, they are not likely to show up on an x-ray, computed tomography (CT) scan, or magnetic resonance imaging (MRI; Difiori & Giza, 2010; Pulsipher, Campbell, Thoma, & King, 2011). Such scans may be run

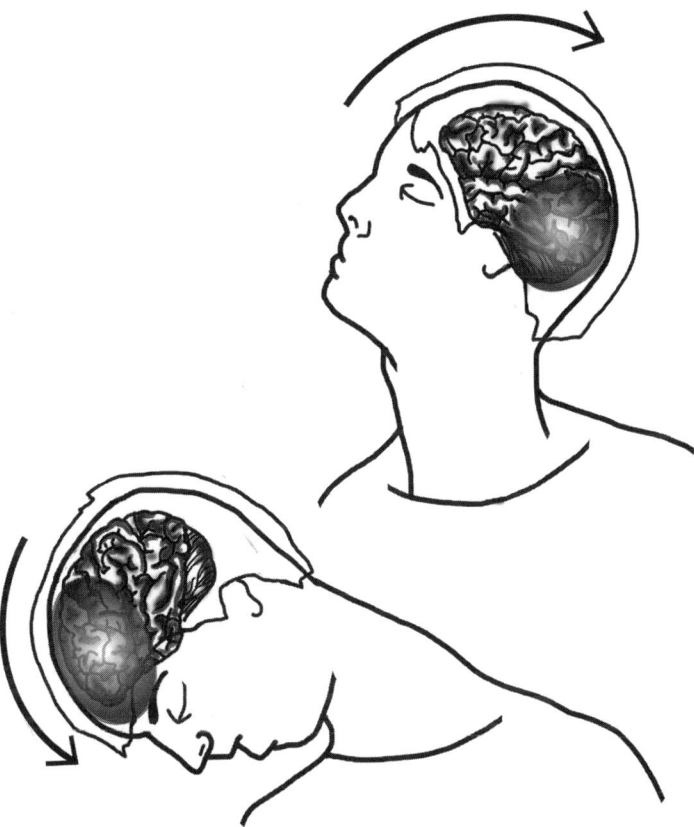

Figure 1.1. Individual sustaining a concussive injury. Courtesy of Maria Tedesco.

to rule out a more serious brain injury, such as intracranial bleeding or contusions, or a skull fracture, but they do not show a concussion. More details on the pathophysiological and neurological effects of a concussion are provided in Chapter 2.

Because they don't show up on typical brain scans or blood tests, concussions can be difficult to diagnose. Currently, concussions are typically identified by observation and reporting of signs and symptoms rather than by a definitive medical test. Thus, if a parent reports that a child's CT scan or MRI was normal, members of the school team should know that this does not eliminate the possibility that there may have been an injury that needs to be treated and monitored.

A number of misnomers have been applied to concussions in the past, many of which minimize our perceptions of their potential dangers. Calling them "bell ringers" or "dings" suggests that they are minor injuries and thus no cause for concern. Therefore it is very appropriate to describe concussions in strict medical terminology—as a type of mild traumatic brain injury. The word *mild*, when coupled with the word *traumatic* conveys more precisely the injury to the brain that has occurred. Less frequently, one might see or hear the terms *head injury* or *head trauma* used when describing a concussive injury; however, these terms can also encompass head injuries that are not concussions, such as skull fractures.

Traumatic brain injuries (TBIs) are typically classified as mild, moderate, or severe, based on scores on the Glasgow Coma Scale (GCS), length of posttraumatic amnesia, and loss of consciousness. Because concussions are mTBIs, they are usually associated with a high GCS (13–15), little or no loss of memory or amnesia, and brief to no loss of consciousness. A 2010 study of high school athletes indicated that only about 5% of their concussions resulted in a loss of consciousness (Meehan, d'Hemecourt, & Comstock, 2010), compared to the 10% that is widely reported based on older studies. In such cases, the loss of consciousness is typically very brief. The classification system of mild–moderate–severe is relatively subjective and is used to reference the severity of the initial trauma; it is not indicative of the long-term consequences of the injury.

PREVALENCE

The Centers for Disease Control and Prevention (CDC, 2014) estimates that in 2010, about 2.5 million ED visits, hospitalizations, or deaths were associated with TBIs. Approximately 75% of these were classified as concussions; however, because many people who sustain concussions do not seek medical treatment, accurate estimates of the prevalence of concussions are difficult to calculate. Taking into account all of the concussions that go unevaluated and undetected, the percentage of brain injuries that could be classified as concussion is likely much higher.

Many of these injuries occur in children—and many are related to sports and recreation activities. Close to 250,000 children in 2009 were treated in U.S. EDs for sports and recreation-related injuries that included a diagnosis of a concussion. Further, from 2001 to 2009, the rate of ED visits for such injuries rose 57% in this age group (Gilchrist et al., 2011). However, again, these statistics do not reflect the numerous concussions that were not treated in an ED or those that went entirely undetected.

Overall, youth from 5 to 18 years of age are at increased risk of experiencing both a TBI and a prolonged recovery (Gilchrist et al., 2011). Within this age group there is a bimodal distribution of TBIs, with incidence rates spiking among preschoolers, largely due to falls, and again in adolescence, largely due to motor vehicle accidents. For adolescents and young adults ages 15 to 24, sports are the second leading cause of TBIs, behind only motor vehicle crashes (Cantu & Hyman, 2012). The likelihood of an athlete in a contact sport (such as football, hockey, or lacrosse) sustaining a concussion may be as high as 20% each season (Cantu & Hyman, 2012).

Data from the National Federation of State High School Associations (NFHS, 2014) Injury Surveillance System indicate that over 140,000 high school athletes across the United States sustain a concussion every year—a number that doesn't even account for nonsports concussion instances or those in younger students. One recent study estimated that nearly 33% of concussions in athletes still go unreported (Meehan, Mannix, O'Brien, & Collins, 2013). This certainly makes tracking injuries and outcomes a complex endeavor.

What do these large numbers about prevalence mean for personnel working in schools? Lewandowski and Rieger (2009) estimate that in a high school of 1,000 students, there is likely to be anywhere from 5 to 10 students per year who experience a concussion. Similarly, Bakhos, Lockhart, Myers, and Linakis (2010) estimated that approximately four in 1,000 children ages 8 to 13 and six in 1,000 children ages 14 to 19 visited the ED for a sports-related concussion.

Incidence rates of TBIs that result in hospitalizations or ED visits are higher in boys than in girls. However, when comparing concussion rates of male and female athletes in high school and college sports, studies found that females had a higher rate of reported concussions (Institute of Medicine & National Research Council, 2014). This may be due in part to physical differences between males and females that make girls more vulnerable to the type of athletic injuries that result in concussions. Because the female neck is not as strong as the male neck, girls' heads move back and forth more quickly upon impact. While neck strengthening exercises may be beneficial, they are not enough to mitigate this increased risk. Furthermore, girls may be more likely to report concussion symptoms than boys.

Discussion related to rates of concussions sustained in sport versus nonsport is also complex. One recent study estimated that about half of concussions seen in U.S. EDs for school-age youth were sports-related concussions; the same study found that approximately 25% of sports-related concussion visits by children 8 to 13 years old occurred during an organized team sport (Bakhos et al., 2010).

However, because many concussions go unreported, this is not a complete data set. It also is difficult to discern what might be categorized as a "sports concussion." Certainly, a concussion sustained in a high school football game would fall squarely in the "sports concussion" category, but there is a continuum of injuries that includes concussions sustained in the following venues:

- School sporting events, such as a middle school soccer match
- Organized school sport practice, such as after-school lacrosse practice
- Nonschool youth athletic leagues, such as Little League Baseball
- Athletic activities, such as a gymnastics class
- Casual sport play, such as baseball in the backyard
- Athletic recreation, such as skateboarding
- General recreation, such as playing on equipment at the playground
- Physical activity, such as dancing in a mosh pit
- Physical engagement, such as fighting

Which of those activities would qualify as a "sports concussion"? As long as different people have different answers to that question, and as long as many concussions go unreported, there will be limited reliable data on the percentage of sport versus nonsport concussions. In the recent publication *Sports-Related Concussions in Youth: Improving the Science, Changing the Culture* (2014), the Institute of Medicine and National Research Council took a broad view of sport, defining it as any sort of vigorous physical activity that did not involve motorized vehicles. Thus, concussions sustained through such activities as playground recreation, physical education class, and ropes courses were included.

CAUSES

School professionals might work with students who sustain concussions from a range of causes, from a preschool student who fell off the monkey bars to a high school student who walked into a pole while texting. The sports and recreation activities associated with most TBI-related ED visits for children age 19 and under are listed in the following order of risks (Gilchrist et al., 2011):

1. Biking
2. Football
3. Playground activities
4. Basketball
5. Soccer
6. All-terrain vehicle riding
7. Skateboarding
8. Swimming
9. Hockey
10. Miscellaneous ball games

Falls are the leading cause of nonsport-related concussions, and they disproportionately affect the youngest and oldest citizens. More than 55% of TBIs of all severity levels among children ages 0 to 14 were caused by falls.

RISK FACTORS

The majority of concussions resolve within 2 to 3 weeks without prolonged complications; however, doctors cannot predict the outcome of a student's concussion at the time of injury. Sometimes, a very forceful blow to the head results in few symptoms and a quick recovery. Other times, a student may sustain what seems to be a relatively mild hit and then have many symptoms for a prolonged period of time. Similarly, a student who initially seems fine may then have delayed symptoms, whereas another student who initially has significant symptoms may recover quickly.

Admittedly, some students are at higher risk for sustaining a concussion than others. These students include athletes, risk-takers, and students who are impulsive. Students who play football and hockey might immediately come to mind when considering sports-related concussions, but virtually every sport poses some degree of risk, including flag-twirling (and flag-dropping) color guard members, the volleyball players who collide and fall on hard surfaces, and the cheerleaders who toss (and, yes, sometimes drop) one another into the air. Swimmers can slip on a pool deck and land on their heads, baseball players can have unfortunate collisions with swinging bats or the opposing team's base players, and divers can crack their heads on the diving board. Ask any physician at a sports concussion clinic for details, and you will likely hear dozens of stories of different concussion cases and outcomes. Once a student sustains a concussion, no matter the sport or circumstances, a number of factors can affect the manifestation of symptoms and the trajectory of recovery.

Other risk factors for more intense symptoms or for protracted recovery include students with a history of previous concussions and those who have a history of migraines/headaches. Similarly, students with a history of learning disabilities, attention deficit hyperactivity disorder (ADHD), or other developmental disorders may also be at higher risk, as are those with sleep disorders or previous mental health problems, including anxiety, depression, and other psychiatric disorders (CDC, 2010). Yet others appear to have no discernible risk factors, but for some unknown reason, they develop persistent post-concussion symptoms.

Childhood as a risk factor

More research is needed, but preliminary data indicate that young children are at particular risk for adverse effects of concussions. Much of this is related to developmental issues. The young brain is underdeveloped when compared to older brains. First, the myelin sheaths in young neurons are not fully formed. Myelin is the fatty tissue that covers the fiber tracts in the brain. Adult neurons are covered with a coating of myelin that protects against injury. Although adult brains can certainly still be damaged, myelin helps defend them against injury. In contrast, young brains have less myelin, leaving them structurally vulnerable to damage.

In addition to neuronal risk, the physical stature of young children also places them at risk for the adverse effects of blows to the head or body. Younger children's heads and brains are proportionally larger when compared to their bodies than those of adults. This proportional matter is particularly pronounced in early childhood. And when combined with the weaker neck of young children—particularly females—this extra size and weight means that a child's head cannot withstand the force of a hit the way a typical adult's can. Some may argue that young children are protected because child-on-child physical forces are not as strong as those sustained in adult-on-adult collisions. However, the force that is transferred to the head may be greater due to these proportional differences. Children also have thinner cranial bones and a larger subarachnoid space in which the brain can move, as well as differences in cerebral blood volume. All of these factors can make them more susceptible to concussions than older individuals (Karlin, 2011).

An additional factor related to childhood risk is simply the increased risk of cumulative trauma. If young football players are engaging in full-body contact drills beginning in early childhood, the sheer number of potential concussive blows increases. Much of the emerging research on postmortem brains of athletes who developed chronic traumatic encephalopathy (CTE), a chronic degenerative brain disorder, indicates that both concussions and subconcussive blows (repeated hits to the head that were not necessarily diagnosed as concussions) can be risk factors.

Adolescence as a risk factor

The risk-taking behaviors among adolescents can put this population at increased risk for concussion. This may be in part because the adolescent prefrontal cortex, the area of the brain that is important in executive decision making, emotion regulation, and risk assessment, continues developing into young adulthood. To complicate the risk even more, today's youth have an earlier average age of puberty when compared with previous generations (Biro et al., 2010). This leads to an interesting mismatch—and essentially a longer than ever time frame—of a propensity toward risk-taking spurred on by both the onset of puberty and by behavioral inhibition due to the developing prefrontal cortex (Institute of Medicine & National Research Council, 2014).

THE UNDERREPORTING OF CONCUSSIONS

Although there is now greater awareness among coaches and players about the dangers of concussions and the need for appropriate treatment, there remains a tendency to underreport known or suspected concussions. The culture, particularly among athletes, resists both self-reporting of concussions and compliance with concussion management plans (Institute of Medicine & National Research Council, 2014). The hesitancy of youth to acknowledge their concussions as "real" injuries is a serious problem.

Students who fail to report concussions can experience subsequent problems with a variety of untreated symptoms (Comper, Hutchison, Richards, & Mainwaring, 2012; Laker, 2011; Lewandowski & Rieger, 2009), including problems related to physical activity, cognitive ability, emotional regulation, and sleep (Halstead & Walter, 2010). Because concussions are not visible injuries, athletic and medical professionals heavily depend on the individual to self-report suspected concussions (Mainwaring, Hutchison, Comper, & Richards, 2012). Therefore, students—particularly student athletes—need to be repeatedly informed about concussion symptoms, possible consequences, and the importance of immediately reporting concussion signs and symptoms.

Of course, even when student athletes *are* better educated about concussions, they often fail to report them. The problem of underreporting of concussion is not well understood. A recent study, however, identified a number of reasons why college athletes failed to report known or suspected concussions (Davies & Bird, 2015). Critical barriers to reporting included not wanting to be pulled out of a game, not wanting to let down their team, and thinking that the injury was just not serious enough. These findings were similar to a 2004 study in which a large sample of high school football players from 20 schools revealed that they reported only about 47% of their concussions even though 30% had a previous history of concussion. In this study, the most common reasons for not reporting concussions were not thinking the injury was serious enough to warrant medical attention, not wanting to be withheld from competition, and lack of awareness of probable concussion (McCrea, Hammeke, Olsen, Leo, & Guskiewicz, 2004).

Clearly, educating youth about signs and symptoms of concussion is important, but education alone is not sufficient to address the problem. Many athletes know the signs and symptoms of concussion—and the potential for additional injury during recovery—yet they frequently choose not to report concussion symptoms to a coach or athletic trainer. Overall, there is a culture of resistance to reporting concussions. To add to this difficulty, concussions are often not appropriately diagnosed in the hospital. De Maio et al. (2014) found that of 218 children age 6 to 18 who met the Third International Conference on Concussion in Sport diagnostic criteria for concussion (McCrory et al., 2009), the majority were treated and released from a level 1 trauma center ED without a concussion-specific diagnosis or activity restrictions. Thus, school personnel should be aware that a student who sustained a significant blow to the head who is presenting with postconcussion symptoms—even without a diagnosis from the ED—may require adjustments and monitoring at school. In such cases, they should refer the family to a medical specialist with experience in concussion evaluation and management.

It is important that school personnel seek to clarify and address factors related to the intention of underreporting known and suspected concussions. They can also specifically address the concerns about reporting concussions that were identified in the two research studies described earlier. School personnel can also focus on the creation of a caring, informed community around school children and adolescents. Finally, it is also important to evaluate how individual student variables, such as the sport played, personal demographics, and so forth, may influence responsiveness to efforts intended to change the culture related to concussions.

Once again, because concussions are invisible injuries, they may be easier to ignore than a gash or a broken bone. However, just like torn ligaments or sprained ankles, concussions require care and attention through the recovery process. Overall, a new attitude needs to be adopted that views concussions as serious injuries requiring care and attention at home, at school, and on the athletic field.

CONCUSSION MYTHS AND MISCONCEPTIONS

In aiming for a truer understanding of concussions, it is helpful to understand what they are *not*. Concussions are not "dings," or "bell-ringers," or minor injuries. They are mTBIs that can have serious repercussions if not treated appropriately. A few more concussion myths must be dispelled. Several of these myths have some grounding in truth, but the distortion of fact has led to many misconceptions.

"If you didn't lose consciousness, you can't have a concussion." This myth may be perpetuated because the first questions asked in cases of head trauma often are, "Did he lose consciousness?" or "Was she knocked out?" In fact, fewer than 10% of concussions likely resulted in any loss of consciousness. And even in these cases, the loss of consciousness was likely transient—occurring for less than a minute.

"Concussions that result in loss of consciousness are always more severe than those that do not." While loss of consciousness is an important facet of a head injury that should be documented and considered, it is not *always* the case that a concussion that knocks someone out is more serious than one that does not. Again, every concussion is different.

"If someone doesn't have symptoms right away, it's not a concussion." Concussion symptoms often are present immediately—but not always. For example, Kevin, age 13, was in a fight over the weekend. He ended up with a number of cuts and bruises, which he had treated at a local urgent care center. Back at school on Monday, however, Kevin complained of fatigue and difficulty concentrating and reading. Over the weekend, he rested and did not really need to concentrate or read. It was only when mental focus and cognitive exertion were required that his concussion symptoms became apparent.

"A child vomiting after a blow to the head means they had a concussion." Although vomiting can be a sign of concussion, a child's being scared or shocked after an incident can also be a cause for vomiting. For instance, Matthew was sitting on a tree branch that broke and he fell to the ground. His mother came out of the house screaming. Matthew jumped up, cried, and vomited. The incident was awful and terrifying for Matthew and his mother, but he had no broken bones, no cuts, and no concussion. Yet, along with other symptoms—severe headache, confusion, and dizziness—vomiting can certainly indicate the possibility of concussion or an even more severe injury. It is an important sign of concussion, but does not automatically mean someone has sustained a concussion.

"You have to get hit in the head to have a concussion." A number of concussions occur without a direct blow to the head. Concussions can also be sustained from a blow to the body that in turn causes the head to whip and the brain to shift inside the skull. In fact, many concussions from football tackles occur this way. The brain can scrape or bang against the ridged surface inside the skull and neurons can be stretched and sheared to the point of injury. These forces can cause a concussion without a direct hit to the head.

"Helmets prevent concussions." Helmets offer important protection against skull fractures and head lacerations. They are required gear in collision sports because they protect against focal blows in which force is concentrated in a small area. In some cases, they can help minimize the effect of a potentially concussive blow to the head. For example, in hockey, a player's helmet can help protect the skull from an opponent's swinging stick or the flying puck. The helmet's hard casing is designed to spread the force of the blow over a wider area, thereby dampening the force and reducing the chance of concussion.

Holly, for example, was a hockey player who sustained such an injury. She had been playing for several years and was in her final game of the season. As Holly went after the puck at the end of the first period, an opponent also swung for the puck. The opponent's stick hit the side of Holly's helmet with significant force. In Holly's case, the helmet not only reduced risk of concussion, it also significantly reduced the risk of a hematoma, or bleeding, in her brain, while protecting her from a skull fracture.

However, in another hockey incident, Gabe was skating at full speed when he collided with another player and fell on the ice. In this instance, the helmet provided much less protection against concussion. That is because in such a case, the whipping action of Gabe's head and the acceleration force stressed his brain—the brain hitting against the *inside* of his skull caused the damage. The helmet offers little protection against this type of hit.

"My child's CT scan and MRI were clear, so he did not have a concussion." Generally neither CT scans nor MRIs can detect concussions. Hospitals typically administer these scans because they are looking for different types of injuries, such as bleeding or fractures. For the time being, the only way to find out whether or not a child sustained a concussion is through reporting of symptoms. In cases of very young children, who do not yet have the language to describe how they are feeling, it can be more difficult to determine whether they had a concussion. In these cases, physicians are looking more at observable signs and depending on reports from parents. Some computerized tests that measure reaction time and memory, such as ImPACT, which is discussed in Chapter 4, can also aid in the diagnosis of concussion, as long as there is also a baseline assessment of how the child performed on such a test prior to his or her injury.

"The harder the hit, the worse the concussion." There is not always a direct correlation between the strength of the concussive blow and the intensity or duration of symptoms. The child's age, physical condition, pre-existing conditions, and other variables can all factor into recovery.

"All concussions have the same set of symptoms." While headache and confusion are commonly reported, it is important to keep in mind that no two concussions are alike. Some students will seem irritable and have difficulty sleeping. Others will have trouble concentrating or reading. If a teacher has had one student recovering from a concussion while in class, the teacher should not expect the next student to present the same way or to recover at the same rate. Individual symptoms and categories of symptoms will be discussed in detail later in this book.

"Concussions are a bigger problem for boys than girls." As discussed in the "Prevalence" section, there are gender differences in concussions, but it is not as simple as being "worse" for one gender than for the other. Once again, symptoms can vary between genders. One study of high school athletes indicated females reported more somatic symptoms, such as drowsiness and sensitivity to noise, while boys reported more cognitive symptoms, including amnesia, confusion, and disorientation (Frommer et al., 2011). Girls may also be more likely to report their symptoms.

One 2007 study found that: (a) concussion rates in high school soccer were 68% higher for girls than for boys, (b) concussion rates in high school basketball were three times higher for girls than for boys, and (c) recovery time for girls was longer than for boys (Gessel, Fields, Collins, Dick, & Comstock, 2007). A later study yielded similar results, finding that in gender-comparable sports such as soccer and basketball, girls had a higher concussion rate than boys (Marar, McIlvain, Fields, & Comstock, 2012).

This issue may not be as straightforward as simply more girls than boys sustain concussions in these sports. It may be the case that athletic trainers pay more attention to girls' signs and symptoms than to boys', pulling them out of the game more readily and essentially protecting female participants more than males. Perhaps culture is a factor and boys are more encouraged to be tough and to shrug off injuries. Perhaps the varying numbers can be partially attributed to differences in training, whereby boys are better trained to handle the blows. Finally, as mentioned previously, a significant variable is likely the differences in body types, with boys having bigger and stronger necks than girls. The bottom line is that gender is a complex issue in terms of concussion rates and reporting.

"Concussions aren't as bad for younger kids because their sports aren't as rough" or **"Concussions aren't as bad for younger**

kids because their brains can bounce back more easily." As described earlier, young children are uniquely vulnerable to the risk associated with head trauma. The young brain is still developing and it may take young children longer to recover from concussions.

"After three concussions, an athlete should stop playing sports altogether." While multiple concussions may certainly contribute to the presence of persistent symptoms, there is no magic number that should determine the course of one's athletic career. Thus, in addition to the number of concussions, students, their parents, and their physicians should consider other factors, including the severity of each concussion, the length of time between concussions, the force of the concussive blows, and the constellation of concussion symptoms. For example, after sustaining one concussion in elementary school, 15-year-old Elise fell on the pool deck and sustained a blow to the head of minor force. The injury resulted in a complex and persistent constellation of concussion symptoms, which may indicate that Elise has a low threshold for head trauma, an indication that needs to be taken very seriously. Elise had previously played on her school's lacrosse team, but after her concussion, she and her family decided she would instead pursue her love of piano and art.

"Mouthguards prevent concussion" and **"Sports headbands prevent concussion."** Mouthguards can protect the mouth during sports, and headbands can keep players' hair out of their eyes, but they don't prevent concussions. See the discussion on protective gear in Chapter 7.

"Most concussions in children are caused by football." According to the CDC, more children sustain TBIs from biking than from any other activity. Very few girls play tackle football, which skews the numbers. Concussion rates due to football in boys under 10 are also lower than those due to bicycling or playground accidents. Football does, however, top the list of concussion rates in organized sports for children ages 12 to 17 (Ferguson, Green, & Hansen, 2013).

"Parents should wake their child who has had a concussion every 20 minutes." The child or adolescent who is recovering from a concussion should be checked on periodically; however, keeping them awake is not necessary once a more serious brain injury—such as a brain bleed—has been ruled out. In fact, a good night of uninterrupted sleep is one of the best mechanisms of recovery for concussion.

A physician can advise parents on the proper steps to recovery; typically, this will involve plenty of rest. Thus, interrupting this rest may prolong recovery.

CONCUSSION LEGISLATION AND POLICIES

Concussion laws and policies have now been established in all states requiring that a student athlete suspected of having sustained a concussion be removed from play. These policies generally stipulate that a written release from a health care professional is required before a child who has been removed from play due to a head trauma can resume participation in the sport. They also typically include stipulations requiring that athletic coaches complete concussion education sessions.

It is important that all school professionals become familiar with the specific language of the legislation that has been adopted by their home state. For example, each state may have different definitions of who constitutes a qualified health care professional. Furthermore, some districts may have more strict standards than those established by state law. Three tenets of model legislation include the following:

- Education of coaches, officials, parents, and student athletes
- Removal from play if a concussion is reasonably suspected
- Clearance by a licensed health care professional for return to play

These rules typically cover, at a minimum, athletes playing on middle and high school teams. Some states have wisely elected to include legislation that also reaches into private youth sports organizations, such as Little League Baseball and Pop Warner Football. Many state concussion laws also require a gradual re-entry plan for sports with a step-by-step process. These laws often incorporate the "Return to Play" protocol developed at the Third International Conference on Concussion in Sport held in Zurich (McCrory et al., 2009), a protocol that involves a step-wise decision-making process for determining when an athlete is ready to resume practice and game play.

Efforts to develop a similar "Return to Learn" protocol have begun taking root in the past few years (Halstead et al., 2013). Such protocols can help students who return to school while still symptomatic. Upon returning to school, students often require physical, emotional, and academic support. Schools can play a crucial role in facilitating a student's transition back to school postconcussion. Without adequate understanding and support—and policies to require that schools provide this support—students with concussions may experience prolonged symptoms, educational difficulties, and social/emotional/behavioral problems, all of which are discussed in more detail in Chapter 2.

CASE STUDIES

We will follow four students throughout this book. Each child sustained a concussion in a different way, at a different age, and with different outcomes. We will revisit each of these four students at various points. These illustrative case studies can provide useful discussion points for school teams using this book as part of their concussion team training. Although the real-world application of the cases can help make some of the issues more realistic, it is important that educators keep in mind that no set of cases can perfectly encapsulate all of the variables and nuances they might encounter when responding to concussion cases.

Julia

Julia was an eleventh-grade honors student and star athlete; she played both basketball and soccer. At the beginning of the fall semester, she sustained her third concussion in 2 years. Three months later, she continued to suffer from postconcussion symptoms, including headaches, difficulty learning new material, and a low tolerance for frustration.

Damien

Damien was an eighth-grade boy who was in a car accident that resulted in a broken leg, numerous cuts and abrasions, and a concussion. His family, teachers, and medical providers tended to focus first and foremost on his visible injuries. However, he was also struggling with concussion symptoms that made the transition back to school particularly difficult.

Ben

Ben was a fourth grader who played youth football in his community's recreational league. During a weekend game, a player from the opposing league collided with Ben. There was no direct helmet-to-helmet contact, and Ben's head did not hit the ground; therefore, his parents and coach did not think he could have sustained a concussion. However, that evening he was nauseous and, when asked by his mother, Ben said he could not remember the collision.

Carly

Carly was a first-grade student who fell headfirst off the monkey bars on the playground. The playground aide did not see the fall, but she sent her to the office. The school nurse was not in that day. The secretary had Carly lie down for the rest of recess and then sent her back to class. Carly's teacher thought Carly seemed fine and no documentation or phone call home was made. That evening, however, Carly's mother noticed she was acting strangely—she seemed unusually tired and very moody, despite sleeping well the night before. The next day, the bright lights and loud noises at school bothered Carly and she told her teacher she felt dizzy.

REFERENCES

Bakhos, L. L., Lockhart, G. R., Myers, R., & Linakis, J. G. (2010). Emergency department visits for concussion in young child athletes. *Pediatrics, 126*(3), e550–e556. doi:10.1542/peds.2009-3101.

Biro, F. M., Galvez, M. P., Greenspan, L. C., Succop, P. A., Vangeepuram, N., Piney, S. M., ... Wolff, M. S. (2010). Pubertal assessment method and baseline characteristics in a mixed longitudinal study of girls. *Pediatrics, 126*(3):e583–e590. doi:10.1542/peds.2009-3079

Cantu, R., & Hyman, M. (2012). Concussion and our kids: *America's leading expert on how to protect young athletes and keep sports safe.* New York, NY: Houghton Mifflin Harcourt Publishing Company.

Centers for Disease Control and Prevention. (2010). *Heads up: Facts for physicians about mild traumatic brain injury (MTBI).* Retrieved from http://www.cdc.gov/concussion/headsup/pdf/facts_for_physicians_booklet-a.pdf

Centers for Disease Control and Prevention. (2014). *Injury prevention and control: Traumatic brain injury.* Retrived from http://www.cdc.gov/TraumaticBrainInjury/data/index.html

Centers for Disease Control and Prevention. (2015). *Traumatic brain injury in the United States: Fact sheet.* Retrieved from http://www.cdc.gov/traumaticbraininjury/get_the_facts.html

Comper, P., Hutchison, M. G., Richards, D., & Mainwaring, L. (2012). A model of current best practice for managing concussion in university athletes: The University of Toronto approach. *Clinical Journal of Sport Psychology, 6*(3), 231–246.

Davies, S. C., & Bird, B. M. (2015). Motivations for under-reporting suspected concussions in college athletics. *Journal of Clinical Sport Psychology, 9*(2), 101–115. doi:10.1123/jcsp.2014-0037

De Maio, V. J., Joseph, D. O., Tibbo-Valeriote, H., Cabanas, J. G., Lanier, B., Mann, C. H., & Register-Mihalik, J. (2014). Variability in discharge instructions and activity restrictions for patients in ED postconcussion. *Pediatric Emergency Care, 30*(1), 20–25. doi:10.1097/PEC.0000000000000058

Difiori, J. P., & Giza, C. C. (2010). New techniques in concussion imaging. *Current Sports Medicine Reports, 9*(1), 35–39. doi:10.1249/JSR.0b013e3181caba67

Ferguson, R. W., Green A., & Hansen L. M. (2013). *Game changers: Stats, stories and what communities are doing to protect young athletes.* Washington, DC: Safe Kids Worldwide.

Frommer, L. J., Gurka, K. K., Cross, K. M., Ingersoll, C. D., Comstock, R. D., & Salibal, S. A. (2011). Sex differences in concussion symptoms of high school athletes. *Journal of Athletic Training, 46*(1), 76–84. doi:10.4085/1062-6050-46.1.76

Gessel, L. M., Fields, S. K., Collins, C. L., Dick, R. W., & Comstock, R. D. (2007). Concussions among United States high school and collegiate athletes. *Journal of Athletic Training, 42*(4), 495–503.

Gilchrist, J., Thomas, K., Xu, L., McGuire, L., & Coronado, V. (2011). Nonfatal traumatic brain injuries related to sports and recreation activities among persons aged <19 years—United States 2001–2009. *Centers for Disease Control and Prevention Morbidity and Mortality Weekly Report, 60*(39), 1337–1342.

Halstead, M. E., McAvoy, K., Devord, C., Carl, R., Lee, M., Logan, K., ... Council on School Health. (2013). Returning to learning following a concussion. *Pediatrics, 132*(5), 948–957. doi:10.1542/Peds.2013-2867

Halstead, M. E., & Walter, K. D. (2010). Clinical report—sport-related concussion in children and adolescents. *Pediatrics, 126*(3), 597–615. doi:10.1542/peds.2010-2005

Institute of Medicine (IOM) and National Research Council. (2014). *Sports-related concussions in youth: Improving the science, changing the culture.* Washington, DC: The National Academies Press.

Karlin, A. M. (2011). Concussion in the pediatric and adult population: Different population, different concerns. *American Academy of Physical Medicine and Rehabilitation, 3,* S369–S379. doi:10.1016/jpmrj.2011.07.015

Laker, S. R. (2011). Epidemiology of concussion and mild traumatic brain injury. *PM&R, 3,* S354–S358. doi:10.1016/j.pmrj.2011.07.017

Lewandowski, L. J., & Rieger, B. (2009). The role of a school psychologist in concussion. *Journal of Applied School Psychology, 25*(1), 95–110. doi:10.1080/15377900802484547

Mainwaring, L. M., Hutchison, M., Comper, P., & Richards, D. (2012). Examining emotional sequelae of sport concussions. *Journal of Clinical Sport Psychology, 6,* 247–274.

Marar, M., McIlvain, N. M., Fields, S. K., & Comstock, R. D. (2012). Epidemiology of concussions among U.S. high school athletes in 20 sports. *American Journal of Sports Medicine, 40*(4), 747–755. doi:10.1177/036354651143526

McCrea, M., Hammeke, T., Olsen, G., Leo, P., & Guskiewicz, K. (2004). Unreported concussion in high school football players: Implications for prevention. *Clinical Journal of Sports Medicine, 14*(1), 13–17. doi:10.1097/00042752-200401000-00003

McCrory, P., Meuwisse, W., Johnston, K., Dvorak, J., Aubry, M., Molloy, M., & Cantu, R. (2009). Consensus statement on concussion in sport: The 3rd international conference on concussion in sport held in Zurich, November 2008. *Journal of Athletic Training, 4,* 434–444. doi:10.1136/bjsm.2009.058248

Meehan, W. P., III, d'Hemecourt, P., & Comstock, R. D. (2010). High school concussions in the 2008–2009 academic year: Mechanism, symptoms, and management. *American Journal of Sports Medicine, 38*(12), 2405–2409. doi:10.1177/0363546510376737

Meehan, W. P., III, Mannix, R. C., O'Brien, M. J., & Collins, M. W. (2013). The prevalence of undiagnosed concussions in athletes. *Clinical Journal of Sport Medicine, 23*(5), 339–342. doi:10.1097/JSM.0b013e318291d3b3

National Federation of State High School Associations (NFHS) Sports Medicine Advisory Committee. (2014). *A parent's guide to concussion in sports.* Retrieved from http://www.nfhs.org/sports-resource-content/a-parents-guide-to-concussion

Pulsipher, D. T., Campbell, R. A., Thoma, R., & King, J. H. (2011). A critical review of neuroimaging applications in sports concussion. *Current Sports Medicine Reports, 10*(1), 14–20. doi:10.1249/JSR.0b013e31820711b8

CHAPTER 2

The Aftermath: Effects of Concussions

This chapter describes what happens after a concussion, from the immediate changes in neurochemistry to the signs and symptoms that may be present in the days, weeks, and months following the event. The neuropsychological effects, including cognitive, physical, emotional/mood, and sleep symptoms are discussed in depth. Dangers signs are also described, which could be indicative of a more serious brain injury.

Next, there is a discussion of the effects of concussions at different grade levels: elementary school, middle school, high school, and even college. While the clusters of possible signs and symptoms are the same for all age groups, the way they manifest and are acknowledged by students of different ages can vary.

While most concussions dissipate in 2 to 3 weeks, some people experience persistent and prolonged symptoms. Possible long-term effects of concussion are explained in this chapter, including complications associated with multiple concussions, postconcussion syndrome, second impact syndrome, chronic traumatic encephalopathy, and brain injury and suicide.

PATHOPHYSIOLOGICAL AND NEUROLOGICAL CHANGES

Understanding the neurochemistry of a concussion can help students, parents, school personnel, and athletic personnel better understand recovery. It is easy for us to understand lacerations and broken bones because they are injuries visible either to the naked eye or on hospital scans. Students with these injuries return to school with bandages, slings, or casts. However, a concussion is a disruption of neurochemistry—the brain cells become disrupted and imbalanced. While research on the neuroscience behind concussions is still in the early stages—and largely based on animal studies or people with more severe brain injuries—it appears that a series of molecular and functional changes take place in the brain following concussive injuries.

It is believed that after a concussive blow, potassium ions flow out of brain cells and calcium ions flow in, resulting in an inefficiency of brain cells to properly deliver much-needed nutrients (especially glucose) to the brain (Giza & Hovda, 2001). These molecular changes hinder a person's ability to engage in many, if not most, physical or mental activities. Figure 2.1 illustrates a normal, healthy neuronal connection. By contrast, Figure 2.2 depicts a neuron following a concussion and the neurometabolic cascade that disrupts cell functioning.

In the immediate aftermath of a concussion, this dysregulation of brain cells may be so significant that sitting up or keeping one's

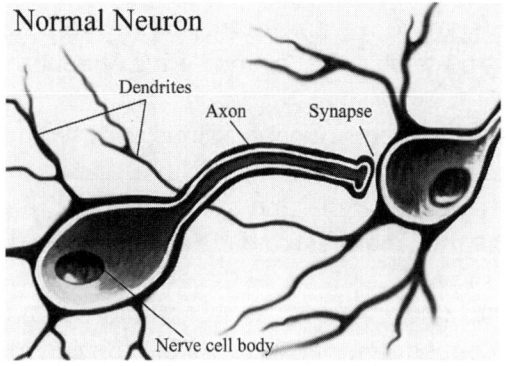

Figure 2.1. Normal neuron. Courtesy of Maria Tedesco.

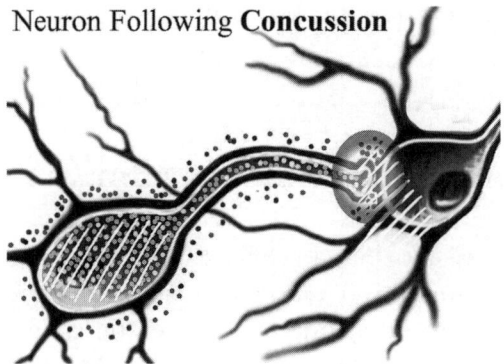

Figure 2.2. Neuron following concussion. This image illustrates the neurometabolic cascade and interrupted communication among neurons. Courtesy of Maria Tedesco.

eyes open is more than the brain can tolerate. This exertion can cause symptoms to flare or be exacerbated (Sady, Vaughan, & Gioia, 2011). This explains why the individual who has sustained a concussion may just want to sleep for the first few days following the injury. Chapter 5 provides more information on the rapid recovery process as cells reregulate in these first hours and days after a concussion.

SIGNS VERSUS SYMPTOMS

In the medical world, *signs* are objectively observable indications of a condition that others can see and report, whereas *symptoms* are subjective features noticed and reported by the patient. Signs and symptoms of concussion are generally evident very soon after the concussive injury. However, some of the signs or symptoms may be delayed; they may not show up for hours or days. Chapter 4 contains assessment tools that can be used in the school to assess the presence and intensity of these signs and symptoms.

Signs of concussion that may be observed by parents or guardians include those listed in Exhibit 2.1 (Centers for Disease Control and Prevention [CDC], 2010).

Symptoms reported by students are organized into four categories: thinking/remembering, physical, emotional, and sleep (Exhibit 2.2; CDC, 2010).

All of these areas can affect learning and schoolwork. For example, cognitive symptoms can affect the ability to learn and

EXHIBIT 2.1

Signs of Concussion Observed by Parents or Guardians

- Appears dazed or stunned
- Is confused about events
- Answers questions slowly
- Repeats questions
- Can't recall events prior to the hit, bump, or fall
- Loses consciousness (even briefly)
- Shows behavior or personality changes
- Forgets class schedule or assignments

EXHIBIT 2.2

Symptoms Reported by Students

Emotional
• Irritable
• Sad
• More emotional than usual
• Nervous
Thinking/Remembering
• Difficulty thinking clearly
• Difficulty concentrating/remembering
• Feeling more slowed down
• Feeling sluggish, hazy, foggy, or groggy
Sleep
• Drowsy
• Sleeps more/less than usual
• Has trouble falling asleep
Physical
• Headache or "pressure" in head
• Nausea or vomiting
• Balance problems or dizziness
• Fatigue or feeling tired
• Sensitivity to light or noise
• Numbness/tingling
• Does not "feel right"

process information, keep track of assignments, and perform well on tests. Physical symptoms can affect a student's focus and concentration. Struggles with school work can further exacerbate the emotional symptoms that were originally caused by changes in brain chemistry. Finally, sleep disturbances can obviously cause fatigue during the school day, further compounding all of the other problem areas.

Concussion symptoms can vary from lasting a few minutes, hours, or days, to weeks, months, or even longer. Some symptoms may not appear immediately after the initial injury, but only after multiple injuries have been sustained. Concussion signs and symptoms differ from person to person; thus, youth who sustain concussions may not experience all symptoms and no single treatment works equally well for all instances of concussion (Aldrich & Obrzut, 2012). Concussion symptoms provide clues related to what is going on in the child's or adolescent's brain. The number and combination of symptoms can indicate which areas of the brain were affected by the concussion. An injury that was focal and isolated to one area may result in fewer, more short-lived symptoms. A more diffuse and widespread injury may result in a greater number of more persistent symptoms.

Symptoms may flare when the brain is asked to do more than it can tolerate. Students who are trying to "tough it out" can make their symptoms worse and prolong recovery. Until they have recovered, students should receive appropriate adjustments or accommodations in all settings, which are discussed later in this book.

Carly (First grade, playground injury)

After school on the day she fell from the monkey bars, Carly went outside to play with her younger brother, Henry. However, after about a half hour, Carly came back inside, saying she "didn't feel good." She went up to her room to lie down.

Later that evening, Carly began her math homework. After a few minutes she started to cry.

"I can't do these!" she shouted.

Her mother looked over Carly's shoulder. "Yes, you can. I saw you do the same type of problems last week. It's nothing new."

"No!" Carly sobbed. "I don't feel good." She covered her eyes with her arms and put her head on the table.

Both the physical and cognitive exertion caused by playing outside and focusing on homework, respectively, can cause symptoms to flare, particularly in the first few days after a concussive injury. Had her parents known she had fallen at recess, they may have taken Carly to be examined by a doctor so her family could get a more definitive diagnosis and recommendations for treatment. A physician would likely have told Carly's parents that she had a concussion. The doctor also would have likely recommended both physical and cognitive rest. In this case, Carly's parents sent her to school the next day, and the teacher reported to the nurse that she suspected Carly had a concussion.

DANGER SIGNS

A student should be taken to the emergency department right away if any of the signs listed in Exhibit 2.3 are observed. The child should be watched carefully, particularly in the first 48 to 72 hours following injury, for any of these signs. The presence of one or more of these "danger signs" may indicate an injury that is more severe than a concussion (CDC, 2010):

Ben (Fourth grade, football injury)

The evening after Ben's tackle during a youth football game, his father asked him about the game.
"It was good," he said. "We won."
"Tell your dad about that major tackle, though," his mother prompted.
"What tackle?" Ben asked.
"When that huge player from the Eagles hit you from the side and you went flying through the air!" his mother exclaimed. "You scared your sister and me to death!"
"Um, I'm not really sure," Ben said.
"It's just a good thing you didn't hit your head," Ben's mother said.
"Did you get back in the game?" Ben's dad asked.
"Oh yeah," Ben said proudly. "I played most of the game."
An hour later, when coming to the dinner table, Ben abruptly sat on the floor, put his head in his hands and moaned.
"Ben, what's the matter?" his mother asked, kneeling down next to him.
"My head really hurts. It kind of hurt before, but now it really, really hurts."

EXHIBIT 2.3
Danger Signs

- One pupil that is larger than the other.
- Drowsiness or inability to wake up.
- A headache that gets worse and does not go away.
- Slurred speech, weakness, numbness, or decreased coordination.
- Repeated vomiting or nausea, convulsions, or seizures (shaking or twitching).
- Unusual behavior, increased confusion, restlessness, or agitation.
- Loss of consciousness (passed out/knocked out). Even a brief loss of consciousness should be taken seriously.

"Aw, sweetie. I'll give you some ibuprofen. Come have some dinner first. I made your favorite spaghetti and meatballs." she said.

"Ugh, I'm not hungry," Ben said. "I feel like I'm going to throw up."

Ben did throw up—several times over the next 2 hours. He seemed "not himself," and he exhibited increased confusion and agitation. Ben's mother called her sister, a nurse, who said Ben should be checked out in an emergency department for a concussion.

Ben's mother took him to the hospital. He received a CT scan and MRI, both of which showed up normal. He was, however, diagnosed with a concussion based on the signs he exhibited and the symptoms he reported.

Ben's aunt offered good advice when she suggested that his mother take him to the hospital right away. Ben was showing some of the danger signs that might have indicated a more serious brain injury. As is evident in Ben's case, the presence of several danger signs—unusual behavior, repeated vomiting, and an increasing headache—does not automatically indicate a severe brain injury, but they are signs that warrant an immediate and complete medical evaluation. In this specific case, although Ben exhibited a couple of the danger signs, he luckily had not experienced a more serious brain injury. He did, however, have a concussion that needed particular care and treatment.

EFFECTS AT DIFFERENT GRADE LEVELS

Elementary school

After a concussion, younger children tend to complain more about physical symptoms than older students. They may describe their head as feeling "like it's being squeezed," their tummy as feeling "yucky," or their body as feeling "tired." They may also act out more when experiencing cognitive overload and fatigue. They may have meltdowns, outbursts, or simply not act like themselves.

Elementary teachers likely have fewer students and typically know their students' parents better than teachers of older students. Therefore, they may have greater responsibility in assisting a concussed student through the recovery process. The parents or teachers might want to talk with the student's classmates to let them know that the signs and symptoms are not contagious and to give them ideas on how they can help and support their friend. Such ideas might include engaging in a quiet activity with the concussed student during recess or helping carry the student's heavy bookbag.

Middle school

Friends and an active social life are increasingly important in middle school. The middle school student might try to hide concussion symptoms so he or she does not stand out or require special attention. Conversely, some middle schoolers may overdramatize symptoms in order to gain attention. As one physician who is a concussion specialist said, "*With a lot of these middle schoolers, [on the 0–6 symptom rating scale] everything was a '6.' Every day they were 'dying' but you know it really wasn't that bad ... but of course you can't say that to them.*"

The transition from elementary school to middle school can be difficult for many students, but particularly for a student who has sustained a concussion. The student may have already been grappling with the increased responsibility for self-management, organization, and planning ahead. The concussion can make these tasks much more difficult. Thus, it is important for the school to communicate clearly with the student, his or her parents, and the student's medical providers so everyone has a clear picture of the student's symptoms and specific areas of difficulty.

Damien (Eighth grade, car accident)

Damien was a bright and successful elementary school student. He easily earned good grades and his teachers generally liked him. The move to middle school was difficult for him. His group of friends were scattered among the students from the five other elementary schools—he almost never saw them. He had to change classes, manage a locker, plan projects and homework, and adjust his behavior and work to meet the expectations of seven different teachers.

By the end of seventh grade, he had it all figured out. He started eighth grade strong. Then he was in the car accident.

Damien not only experienced a concussion, but also a broken leg and lacerations. The night before he returned to school, it took Damien several hours to fall asleep. He had a terrible headache and was filled with anxiety about what to say to people and how to catch up on all the school work he had missed. However, he did not tell his parents how he was feeling and showed up at school the next day.

High school

High school students have moved even further from parents and more toward independence. A concussion can increase the need for parental monitoring and lead to a struggle or rift at home. For example, the effects of concussion can make driving inadvisable for a period of time. High school students may be angry or embarrassed at needing to be driven to school when they previously enjoyed the freedom of driving themselves. Managing the overall demands of high school life—homework, extracurricular activities, college applications, relationships, work—can be particularly challenging for a student who is suffering from the effects of a concussion. Parents and educators can help high school students prioritize their activities and reduce overall cognitive and physical demands. This, in turn, can help reduce symptoms such as fatigue, headache, confusion, irritability, and sleepiness.

High school teachers often work with more than a hundred students each day. It can be understandably difficult to monitor and meet the needs of one student who has sustained a concussion. The team model described in the next chapter gives educators support in this process. The student who seems disorganized, unprepared, and lazy might actually be suffering from a concussion; putting appropriate supports in place can help to minimize those kinds of behaviors.

College

Much of the information discussed in this book can be extended to the college setting. Underreporting of concussions is particularly prevalent in college populations (Kroshus, Baugh, Daneshvar, & Viswanath, 2014) despite the relatively high risk for sustaining concussions (Langlois, Rutland-Brown, & Thomas, 2006).

The level of independence expected by college students is high; however, because of limited experience with self-advocacy and self-care during an illness or injury, college students often do not admit that an injury has occurred. The very nature of a concussion results in impaired self-awareness; therefore, a concussed college student may not even suspect that he or she sustained a concussion. A roommate or residence hall advisor may think the student is simply exhausted or still feeling the effects of a weekend of hard partying. Such students often return to classes and sports prematurely without seeking appropriate help.

The college student who knows he or she sustained a concussion may still not take the appropriate self-care steps because the student is panicked about getting behind in school or doesn't want his or her family to worry. The student might not want to cut back on hours at work or involvement in extracurricular activities. Further, college students may consume alcohol while still symptomatic, thereby putting themselves at increased risk for a second concussion before the first has resolved.

Even though it can be annoying to the high school student to have his or her parents hovering and monitoring symptoms, it can be dangerous for the college student with a concussion to *not* have that level of help and support. College students who have sustained concussions should seek help from their residence hall advisor, campus health services office, and/or office for students with disabilities. This can help ensure the student's health and recovery are being monitored and that appropriate academic adjustments can be put in place during the healing process.

PERSISTENT AND SEVERE DIFFICULTIES

While most concussions heal on their own within 1 to 3 weeks, about 10% to 20% of individuals have persistent symptoms. This highlights the "crux of the [concussion] paradox"—that is, an injury considered mild may still result in lasting negative consequences (Comper, Bisschop, Carnide, & Tricco, 2005, p. 864).

Multiple concussions

Once a student has sustained one concussion, he or she is at three to six times higher risk for sustaining another concussion (Guskiewicz, Weaver, Padua, & Garrett, 2000). Sometimes the second concussive blow occurs with less force and often with a more prolonged and difficult recovery. With multiple concussions comes increased risk of persistent postconcussion symptoms. Concussions that occur in close succession—a second one before the first has resolved completely—can be harder for the brain to overcome and may take longer to heal.

Research on the cognitive and symptomatic outcomes of youth who sustain repetitive head trauma is mixed, but more studies report unfavorable changes than do not (Institute of Medicine & National Research Council, 2014). Although catastrophic results of second injuries are very rare, it is more likely that an overall cumulative risk associated with multiple concussions occurs, particularly when a second concussion is sustained before the first has healed. Risk of multiple injuries is particularly problematic in sports, due to both under-reporting of concussions, as well as premature return to play postconcussion.

Concussions often go unreported because individuals are unaware that an injury has occurred. Some may also consider the injury not severe enough to warrant medical attention. In the sports world, some athletes may deliberately choose to not report their injury because they fear losing their reputation, scholarship, or position on the team. Thus, they may return to the game before they are physically ready to do so (McCrea, Hammeke, Olsen, Leo, & Guskiewicz, 2004). This premature return to play can increase the risk of sustaining a second injury before symptoms of the first have resolved, thereby prolonging recovery.

Postconcussion syndrome

The term *postconcussion syndrome* has been used as a diagnosis for individuals who experience significant, persistent postinjury symptoms; however, the diagnosis is controversial, as it lacks a clear definition or consistent application. The most recent edition of the *Diagnostic and Statistical Manual of Mental Disorders*, Fifth Edition (*DSM-5*; American Psychiatric Association [APA], 2013) does not have the previous edition's (*DSM-IV-TR [APA, 2009]*) entry of a diagnostic definition for "postconcussional disorder." Instead, the *DSM-5* retained the broader "neurocognitive disorder due to traumatic brain injury" classification, which includes the diagnostic criterion of persistence "past the acute post-injury period" (APA, 2013, p. 624). A recent study found that 77% of youth who sustained concussions reported symptoms 1 week postinjury, 32% reported symptoms at 3 weeks, and 15% reported symptoms at 3 months (Eisenberg, Meehan, & Mannix, 2014). Another study found similar numbers at the 3-month mark, with about 13% of children reporting symptoms at 3 months postinjury— and 2% continued to be symptomatic after 1 year (Barlow et al., 2010).

In popular use, the term "postconcussion syndrome" or PCS generally applies to concussions that have symptoms which are severe and unusually long lasting. This often occurs as a result of sustaining multiple concussions or in situations involving a pre-existing medical or psychological issue. PCS is likely to affect:

- Academic work
- Classroom participation
- Behavior
- Relationships
- Extracurricular activities

Sleep issues and depression are common in students with PCS. It is particularly important for school teams to assist students who have PCS; engaging them in school as much as possible without exacerbating symptoms can help mitigate the anxiety and depression that can arise in such cases.

Julia (Eleventh grade, soccer injury)

After sustaining her third concussion in 2 years playing soccer, Julia expected to recover within a couple of weeks, just as she did before. However, after several weeks, Julia still struggled with persistent headaches and nausea. She was lethargic and short tempered. Her parents encouraged her to get back into the swing of school and sports, thinking that a regular routine and exercise would help her feel better. Julia had been an honor student, but now her grades in school were slipping; her mother worried she was jeopardizing her chances at securing a soccer scholarship. Julia's teachers were frustrated at what appeared to be her laziness and increasingly bad attitude.

Three months after sustaining her third concussion, Julia was scheduled to take the SAT college entrance exam. She came out of the exam in tears, complaining that her head hurt so much it felt like it was in a vice. She said she knew she did "terrible" on the exam and went home to bed for the rest of the day.

Julia's parents finally took her to a doctor who specialized in evaluating and treating sports-related concussions. The doctor recommended eliminating cognitively and physically stimulating activities that exacerbated Julia's symptoms, as well as avoiding loud, bright, overstimulating environments and technology. Although this made Julia's social circle shrink further, it helped to alleviate her symptoms.

Julia's parents regretted allowing her to go back to participate in soccer before her concussion symptoms cleared. Instead of missing only a week or two of practice and games, she was sidelined for the rest of the season during her junior year.

Second impact syndrome

Second impact syndrome is another poorly understood diagnosis. This is a potentially life-threatening condition that may result from a second (often minor) blow to the head before recovery from the initial injury has occurred. Second-impact syndrome is a very rare condition in which repeated head trauma results in brain swelling, causing the brain to burst within the confines of the skull, leading to herniation and sometimes even death (Byard & Vink, 2009). Those who survive are almost always severely disabled. Because this condition is very rare, there is little prevalence information and some researchers question its validity as a diagnosis entirely. Cases of second impact syndrome have only been reported in children and adolescents.

During a 13-year period, one research team found 94 cases of second impact syndrome, almost all of which were in high school athletes. About 75% of the cases were athletes who had sustained a pervious concussion during the same season (Cantu & Hyman, 2012). Although 94 is a low number when compared to the approximately 1.1 million youth who play high school football in any given year, most of these deaths could have been prevented. These cases can be particularly devastating for those who are left behind—the coaches who sent the player back into the game, the opponents who may have dealt the final tackle, the parents who consented to participation in the sport, and the teammates who knew that their friend was still suffering from concussion symptoms but returned to the field.

The 2006 case of Zackery Lystedt was one that prompted much of the current legislation that now regulates return to play guidelines in schools. Zackery was a 13-year-old who played linebacker for his middle school football team near Seattle, Washington. Near the end of the first half of a game, his head struck the ground after tackling an opponent. He was returned to the game in the third quarter. Near the end of the game, he was part of a big tackle at the goal line, which secured a victory for his school's team. However, after the second half of the game, Zack collapsed on the field. He was airlifted to a medical center and had surgery to remove the left and right sides of his skull in order to relieve the pressure of his swelling brain (CDC, n.d.).

Physicians later indicated that Zack had suffered from second impact syndrome. A concussion that was sustained earlier in the game was not recognized and he was sent back into the game, where he incurred a second blow to the head that almost killed him. Zack was in a coma for 3 months. He did not speak for 9 months. He did not move an arm or leg for 13 months and was on a feeding tube for 20 months (CDC, n.d.). But he survived.

Three years later, Zack returned to school, and 2 years after that he graduated. He was still confined to a wheelchair, but walked across the stage with a cane to receive his diploma. Zack's physical abilities, speech, and short-term memory remain impaired (Cantu & Hyman, 2012). In 2009, the Washington State legislature passed the Zackery Lystedt Law. The National Football League (NFL) refers to the Lystedt Law as model legislation pertaining to student athlete concussion. As described in Chapter 1, the three key provisions require: (a) education and signing of a concussion information form by coaches, parents/guardians, and athletes; (b) immediate removal from a game of any student suspected of having a concussion; and (c) medical clearance before returning to play from someone with training to recognize signs of concussion.

Chronic traumatic encephalopathy (CTE)

Mike Webster, an offensive lineman for the Pittsburgh Steelers in the 1970s and Pro Football Hall of Fame member, played professional football for 17 seasons. In his position, Webster was continually exposed to head trauma. In 2002, Mike Webster died at the age of 50. In the last years of his life, Webster was homeless, unemployed, deeply in debt, and in the process of divorcing his wife. Initial reports indicated that he had died of a heart attack, but the grim truth was later revealed. An autopsy showed damage in the frontal lobe of his brain. It is believed that this damage affected Webster's thinking and reasoning abilities, as well as his attention and concentration, to such an extent that it incapacitated him. The pathologist who examined Webster's brain, Dr. Bennet Omalu, asserted that a contributing factor to Webster's death was chronic traumatic encephalopathy (CTE), a progressively degenerative brain disease that was previously only seen in boxers.

Dr. Omalu also found CTE in Terry Long, another deceased player who played for the Steelers, and who committed suicide by drinking antifreeze. Dr. Omalu believed that Long's erratic behavior and depression toward the end of his life were linked to his diseased brain cells. The reaction to these findings was—and still is—quite controversial. The NFL had three scientists affiliated with the league write letters to a peer-reviewed journal demanding a retraction of Dr. Omalu's published findings. Dr. Omalu's story is at the center of a 2015 motion picture, *Concussion*, starring Will Smith.

CTE has been found postmortem in a number of football players since Dr. Omalu's initial findings, including Junior Seau and Dave Duerson, both of whom committed suicide. Much is yet to be learned about CTE. What is known is that it is found in the brains of some people who have been exposed over many years to repetitive brain trauma, including concussions and subconcussive blows, which are repetitive hits not diagnosed or suspected as concussions. These jolts to the brain can trigger the buildup of tau—an abnormal and toxic form of protein—in brain cells. The process appears similar to that which takes place in the brains of individuals who develop Alzheimer's disease. As the disease progresses, deposits of tau clog neural pathways and damage axons in the brain.

The medial temporal lobe is often affected in such cases, which causes victims to experience impaired functioning in memory and impulse control. Individuals can become depressed and have panic attacks. As the disease progresses, individuals afflicted with CTE may develop violent behavior. Their personal relationships can suffer irreparable damage.

Much remains to be learned about CTE, particularly because the disease can only be diagnosed after death, when the brain is sliced and examined under a microscope. Studies are underway that examine the use of biomarkers and advanced neuroimaging with the hope that there might soon be a reliable way of diagnosing CTE in living individuals. There is currently no treatment for CTE, and no way to slow the progression of the disease. At this point, the cause of CTE seems to be total brain trauma—not just a single concussion; therefore researchers are interested in learning more about the physical impact of the lighter slams and bangs—those multiple subconcussive blows—that are sustained by children who play collision sports. With practices and games, some children might sustain more than a thousand subconcussive blows in a single season, accumulating tens of thousands across their entire athletic career.

The recent discourse about CTE in adult professional athletes certainly has implications for our student populations. Seeing the potential of brain disease that athletic heroes can carry for the rest of their lives can lead to second thoughts when parents are deciding whether or not to sign up their young children for football. While CTE has not been named as the cause of death in adolescent athletes, there have been cases of early stages of CTE being identified in the brains of high school-age athletes, including athletes who have died of second impact syndrome and suicide (Cantu & Hyman, 2012). This raises concerns about the possibility that repetitive brain trauma sustained in collision sports can start the process that results in CTE. And while this alone is not reason to do away with such sports entirely, it certainly is a good reason to consider changing some aspects of youth sports to make them safer, such as eliminating daily full-contact workouts for football players.

Brain injury and suicide

In some cases, the effects of concussions are so intense, and individuals become so distraught, that they become suicidal. Such students must be taken seriously and evaluated by an outside professional, such as a psychiatrist. The association between brain injury and suicide may be in part due to the unrelenting symptoms. The loss of things that are important to the individual—school, sports, cognitive abilities, previously enjoyed freedoms—can also be devastating.

In 2014, Kosta Karageorge, an Ohio State University football player, went missing after he left his mother a note that concussions had his head all messed up. He was soon found dead in a dumpster near his apartment with an apparent self-inflicted gunshot wound. Karageorge was also a wrestler, and his family cited his multiple sports-related concussions as contributing to the depression and confusion that may have led to his suicide (Oster, 2014).

Two years earlier, Jovan Belcher, a linebacker for the Kansas City Chiefs shot and killed his girlfriend and then himself. He was 25 years old and was diagnosed with CTE postmortem. Two years before that, a University of Pennsylvania football player, Owen Thomas, killed himself in his apartment and was later diagnosed with early stages of CTE. These cases represent some of the younger players to demonstrate links between concussions and suicide—a number of older players also committed suicide and were later diagnosed with CTE.

Warning signs that may assist in screening for suicide risk in patients with TBI are listed in Exhibit 2.4. Epidemiological research in the United States found that people with traumatic brain injury (TBI) of all severity levels had an 8% lifetime rate of suicide attempts compared with 2% of population as a whole (Simpson & Tate, 2007).

EXHIBIT 2.4

Warning Signs to Assist Screening for Suicide Risk in Patients With TBI

- Depression/hopelessness
- Relationship breakdown
- Pressure of multiple stressors
- Relationship conflict
- Relationship isolation
- Global impact of injury

• • •

Because the effects of a concussion can vary tremendously from person to person, symptom clusters and recovery rates also vary. Thus, it is important that educators know how to evaluate these symptoms and safely return students to the learning environment and any physical activities. Students who receive academic adjustments in school do so because they are still experiencing effects of a concussion—symptoms are still present. Students who are symptomatic should not resume physical activity. This can be a complicated decision-making process, particularly when a student has several teachers, coaches, and medical providers. A school-based concussion team can help streamline this process. The next chapter provides information to help such teams get started.

REFERENCES

Aldrich, E. M., & Obrzut, J. E. (2012). Assisting students with a traumatic brain injury in school interventions. *Canadian Journal of School Psychology, 27,* 291–301. doi: 10.1177/0829573512455016.

American Psychiatric Association. (2009). *Diagnostic and statistical manual of mental disorders* (4th edition, text revision). Arlington, VA: American Psychiatric Publishing.

American Psychiatric Association. (2013). *Diagnostic and statistical manual of mental disorders* (5th ed.). Arlington, VA: American Psychiatric Publishing.

Barlow, K. M, Crawford, S., Stevenson, A., Sandhu, S. S., Belanger, F., & Dewey, D. (2010). Epidemiology of postconcussion syndrome in pediatric mild traumatic brain injury. *Pediatrics, 126,* e374–e381. doi:10.1542/peds.2009-0925.

Byard, R. W., & Vink, R. (2009). The second impact syndrome. *Forensic Science, Medicine, and Pathology, 5,* 36–38. doi:10.1007/s12024-008-9063-7.

Cantu, R. & Hyman, M. (2012). *Concussion and our kids: America's leading expert on how to protect young athletes and keep sports safe.* New York, NY: Houghton Mifflin Harcourt Publishing Company.

Centers for Disease Control and Prevention. (n.d.). *The Lystedt Law: A concussion survivor's journey.* Retrieved from http://www.cdc.gov/media/subtopic/matte/pdf/031210-Zack-story.pdf

Centers for Disease Control and Prevention. (2010). *Know your concussion ABCs—A fact sheet for school nurses. Heads up to schools: School nurses.* Retrieved from http://www.cdc.gov/headsup/schools/nurses.html

Comper, P., Bisschop, S. M., Carnide, N., & Tricco, A. (2005). A systematic review of treatments for mild traumatic brain injury. *Brain Injury, 19*(11), 863–880. doi:10.1080/02699050400025042.

Eisenberg, M. A., Meehan, W. P., & Mannix, R. (2014). Duration and course of post-concussive symptoms. *Pediatrics, 133,* 999–1006. doi:10.1542/peds.2014-0158.

Giza, C. C., & Hovda, D. A. (2001). The neurometabolic cascade of concussion. *Journal of Athletic Training, 36*(3), 228–235.

Guskiewicz, K. M., Weaver, N. L., Padua, D. A., & Garrett, W. E. Jr. (2000). Epidemiology of concussion in collegiate and high school football players. *The American Journal of Sports Medicine, 28*(5), 643–650.

Institute of Medicine (IOM) and National Research Council. (2014). *Sports-related concussions in youth: Improving the science, changing the culture.* Washington, DC: The National Academies Press.

Kroshus, E., Baugh, C. M., Daneshvar, D. H., & Viswanath, K. (2014). Understanding concussion reporting using a model based on the theory of planned behavior. *Journal of Adolescent Health, 54,* 269–274. doi:10.1016/j.jadohealth.2013.11.011.

Langlois, J. A., Rutland-Brown, W., & Thomas, K. E. (2006). *Traumatic brain injury in the United States: Emergency department visits, hospitalizations, and deaths.* Atlanta, GA: Centers for Disease Control and Prevention, National Center for Injury Prevention and Control.

McCrea, M., Hammeke, T., Olsen, G., Leo, P., & Guskiewicz, K. (2004). Unreported concussion in high school football players: Implications for prevention. *Clinical Journal of Sports Medicine, 14*(1), 13–17. doi:10.1097/00042752-200401000-00003.

Oster, E. (2014, December 16). Do concussions lead to suicide? *FiveThirtyEight.* Retrieved from: http://fivethirtyeight.com/features/do-concussions-lead-to-suicide

Sady, M. D., Vaughan, C. G., & Gioia, G. A. (2011). School and the concussed youth: Recommendations for concussion education and management. *Physical Medicine and Rehabilitation Clinics of North America*, 22(4), 701–719. doi:10.1016/j.pmr.2011.08.008.

Simpson, G. K., & Tate, R. L. (2007). Preventing suicide after traumatic brain injury: Implications for general practice. *Medical Journal Australia*, 187(4), 229–232.

CHAPTER 3

The Concussion Team Model

When any health issue affects a student, school personnel are expected to communicate effectively with one another, with the family, and with medical personnel. Whereas a number of medical situations, such as a student's chronic illness, might develop over time, a concussion occurs in an instant and requires a knowledgeable group of individuals in the school building—with a designated leader—who can quickly and efficiently mobilize to meet the student's needs. A multidisciplinary team approach is best practice in concussion management (Halstead et al., 2013; McAvoy, 2011; Sady, Vaughan, & Gioia, 2011).

This chapter describes the overall structure of a concussion team, as well as a logical delegation of roles. Rather than learning an entirely new skill set, this process largely requires that school personnel tap into their existing skills—and do the types of things they're already doing in their jobs—to assist this specific population of students. This chapter highlights the importance of identifying a concussion team leader (CTL)—one person in the building who is responsible for facilitating the concussion team. This person takes the lead in case consultation, educating the school community about the process, and family–school–medical team collaboration. This chapter also includes a discussion of maintaining student privacy through following Family Educational Rights and Privacy Act (FERPA) and the Health Insurance Portability and Accountability Act of 1996 (HIPAA) regulations. Finally, it concludes with a reminder to consider how the concussion team model can be created in a way that is sustainable across the school years.

THE CONCUSSION TEAM

The presence of a collaborative team can facilitate coordinated, medically approved, return-to-activity decisions. The team can share information related to the student's concussion and observations of the student during the school day. School-based personnel can collaborate with the family to develop an appropriate program that will meet the student's needs. The team can also help explain the plan and rationale for academic adjustments to other school personnel. Additionally, the team is responsible for ongoing assessment of the student's symptoms and progress toward healing.

A district-wide written policy should clarify procedures. This can help ensure continuity in the processes as team members come and go due to job changes. The core concussion team can ensure that all stakeholders in an individual student's situation—including the parents and teachers who may not have extensive training or deep understanding of potential implications of concussions—understand the increased risk of further concussions. The team also ensures that multiple people are watching and helping the student. This team helps determine appropriate adjustments to the educational environment and helps inform *return-to-school* and *return-to-play* decisions.

Damien

When Damien returned to school, he still had visible injuries from his car accident, including a broken leg. Because he had a visible injury, his team of teachers at the junior high knew that he needed special attention and accommodations. He left classes a few minutes early to avoid the rush of people in the hallways, and a classmate assisted by carrying his books. Damien was given extra time to make up the assignments he had missed during his absence and he received a great deal of sympathy and support from both his teachers and his classmates.

However, the staff at Damien's school did not know much about concussions and they did not have a concussion team. Further, because Damien was not an athlete, there was no coach, trainer, or athletic director managing a return-to-play protocol.

Damien did not participate in physical education (PE) class because of his broken leg. During his usual PE period, he went to study hall to catch up on missed work—and there was a lot of it. Because he missed school immediately following his car accident, Damien had fallen far behind on his schoolwork. This included pages of math requiring processes he had never been taught and was trying to figure out on his own. In addition to this extra study hall time at school, Damien was spending hours on homework each night, both trying to catch up and trying to keep on-pace with the new assignments and lessons that were coming his way each day. The homework made his head hurt and sometimes even made his heart race with anxiety. Damien's older brother, Michael, had been driving carelessly and caused the car accident that hurt Damien. Now their parents were upset with Michael and overprotective of Damien. Damien thought the last thing they needed was to hear that he was struggling at school. Damien felt like he was drowning, but he did not say anything to his parents—he did not say anything to anyone.

Once Damien's bandages and cast were removed, everyone was relieved and expected him to be fine. Although Damien was diagnosed with a concussion while in the hospital, both he and his parents thought it was no big deal—that it was the least of his injuries.

Damien's teachers were frustrated that he was not keeping up on his school work. His parents scolded him for being lazy and moody. His brother, Michael, accused him of "milking" the extra attention. Damien's grades started to decline and his friends, who had initially been supportive following the accident, contacted him less and less.

Damien clearly needed a support team at school. A CTL who was aware of the symptoms of concussion could have ensured that appropriate school-based supports were put in place not only for his visible injuries, but also for his invisible concussion. The team could have secured a release of information to talk freely with Damien's medical providers to obtain sound recommendations for helping him at school. They may have suggested that the study hall period be used for resting rather than for catching up on schoolwork without help—which likely required cognitive exertion that exacerbated his symptoms. The team might have collaboratively designed a plan that allowed Damien to be excused from some of his assignments without penalizing him with lowered grades. This kind of accommodation could have helped decrease his anxiety and prevented his headaches and other symptoms from worsening.

The team could also have been a source of much-needed support for Damien's family. They were dealing not only with Damien's injuries, but also with struggles within their family related to his older brother's careless driving. There was arguing, fear, and blaming within Damien's family. While the school-based concussion team is not expected to serve in the role of family therapist, it can be an important source of support for the family. It can be tremendously reassuring to the parents to know that educators are "watching out" for their child and implementing appropriate educational accommodations to meet their child's short- and long-term needs.

TEAM STRUCTURE

Figure 3.1 illustrates the groups of individuals that can comprise an effective concussion team, followed by suggested key members of a concussion team and a description of each team member's potential roles and responsibilities. All of these team members are encouraged to seek out continued professional development regarding concussions.

The family

- ***Parents and Guardians:*** Parents need to be both providers and recipients of information; clear communication with

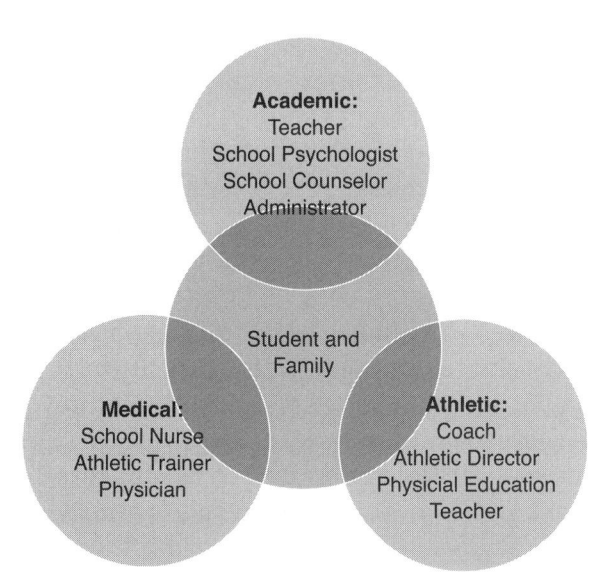

Figure 3.1. Composition of a school-based concussion team. Adapted from Nationwide Children's Hospital (2012a).

medical providers and school personnel is essential. Parents should submit information and instructions from physicians to the school and help their child maintain compliance with recommendations from the medical and academic teams. They should become familiar with their school district's policy and protocol related to return to school and return to academics. Parents know their children best and are often excellent informants of how their child is "different" following a concussion. Thus, parents are important monitors of their child's health during the recovery process and the transition back to a learning environment. They should report any concerns to their child's physician and to the school and follow recommendations from the medical provider related to what the child should and should not be doing at home. Team members can assist parents and guardians by ensuring that they know what a concussion is, the possible effects visible in school, and the importance of following medical guidance.

- ***Student:*** Students should participate in the concussion team process to a degree that is developmentally appropriate. They should follow instructions from their medical provider and be made aware of the risks associated with doing too much too soon. Students who have sustained concussions can share with their parents and other concussion team members what symptoms are most bothersome, which ones are getting better, and their perceptions of how things are going with the accommodation plan. The information provided by students is essential in helping the team support the transition back to regular activities. Thus, students should be encouraged to ask for help and to let teachers know if they are having difficulty with symptoms or assignments. They can use a symptom log (e.g., rate symptoms 0–6 to identify severity). Such a log helps track if symptoms are getting better and can help the school and medical team with the treatment and return to academics process. In more general terms, students can receive education on how to prevent future head injuries, can learn how to recognize signs and symptoms of concussions, and can encourage teammates and classmates to report known or suspected concussions. This can help to change the culture surrounding concussions toward one where concussion reporting is not only acceptable, but encouraged.

Academic team members

- *Teachers:* Teachers can help ensure that students are getting the best education possible and follow recommended academic adjustments. Teachers must refer students suspected of having a concussion—for example, one who states he or she had a bad fall the night before and now appears distracted, sluggish, and confused—to the school nurse or other designated personnel to be evaluated for a suspected concussion. After a student is diagnosed with a concussion, his or her teachers are essential for observing the student's symptoms and recovery trajectory. Teachers are also responsible for implementing appropriate academic adjustments, per the medical provider and/or school concussion team's recommendations. They may also interact regularly with the injured student's parents and report daily changes in the student.

- *School Psychologist:* The school psychologist can evaluate the student's current level of functioning, identify appropriate resources, and facilitate the provision of services. He or she can also assist with ongoing assessment, intervention, and progress monitoring toward a student's recovery. This may include supporting teachers in monitoring the efficacy of specific academic or environmental adjustments that are part of the student's return-to-learn plan. The school psychologist can ensure that students diagnosed with concussions do not substitute mental activities for physical ones unless the medical provider has provided written clearance for the student to do so. The school psychologist may be a consultant for prolonged or complicated cases where long-term adjustments or more extensive assessment and educational plans are required. The school psychologist can also assist in training staff about concussion; he or she can teach the signs and symptoms of a concussion and how a concussion may affect a student in school.

- *School Counselor:* The school counselor can help create and disseminate guidelines regarding academic adjustments to the educational team. The school counselor can provide emotional support for both the student and his or her family. After a student's concussion, parents may become overprotective and restrict previously enjoyed freedoms, such as driving, climbing on equipment, riding bikes, or "rough and tumble" play. All team members—but particularly the school counselor—can listen, validate parents' feelings and concerns, and work toward finding common solutions and goals. The school counselor also might serve as the CTL, particularly if the building does not have a nurse or if the school psychologist is only in the building on a part-time basis.

- ***Administrator:*** The school administrator on the concussion team is responsible for ensuring that there is a concussion management team in place; the administrator is also typically responsible for appointing a CTL. The administrator ensures that the district and building-level policies related to concussion management are implemented and followed. This includes ensuring that the concussion management policy is communicated to school staff. The administrator should also coordinate professional development sessions related to concussion management for staff and parents. When a student sustains a concussion, the administrator can help ensure there is coordination of team efforts and that communication among team members is adequate. Further, the administrator can ensure that educators are supported in their provision of supports and services, including excusals from assignments and assessments, schedule adjustments, grade adjustments (working with teachers to complete grade cards and determine on what work grades should be based), and return-to-play guidelines for student athletes. The administrator can provide guidance to staff members on policies and procedures related to emergency care and transportation of students who may have sustained a concussion. For example, if a student is injured at an after-school practice and the parents cannot be reached, the administrator would need to ensure there is a policy in place and clear understanding among staff members about how such situation are managed. Administrators are key team members in encouraging parents to report concerns about their children to appropriate staff members; they should also encourage parents to communicate with medical providers regarding a time frame for any injured child's return to school. This professional would also be responsible for troubleshooting problems.

- ***Other Academic Personnel:*** Depending on the school, other academic personnel may have significant involvement with the concussion team. For example, speech language pathologists (SLPs) can help monitor students with concussion and identify changes in how a student is communicating or interacting with others. SLPs might assess students and/or give teachers classroom-based strategies to facilitate students' expressive and receptive communication. School secretaries might be the first people to see students with concussions stumble into the office after falling during recess. They need to know what to do in such situations to ensure the student receives prompt and appropriate attention. School social workers might serve in much of the same capacity as school counselors.

Medical team members

- *Physician (or other medical personnel):* The child's physician can describe the injury, severity, and prognosis to the other team members. The physician can also give recommendations and help guide removal of academic supports that may have been part of the recovery process. Because medical providers are governed by HIPAA and school districts are governed by FERPA (see the "Student Privacy" section later in this chapter for more information), it is essential that appropriate releases of information be signed from the outset of the collaboration process to allow bidirectional communication between educators and the medical provider. The medical provider should describe specific symptoms that family members and school personnel should watch out for. He or she should provide a written return-to-activity protocol to follow, or endorse the use of a district-specific return-to-activity schedule. This professional is also typically responsible for providing written clearance for a student athlete to return to play and full activities, including PE class and recess. Teams should clarify their district or state's qualifications for a medical provider to provide this evaluation.
- *School Nurse:* If a child is injured at school, the school nurse will likely be the person to provide an assessment of whether that student is suspected of having sustained a concussion. This will involve a symptom assessment, an observation for signs, and a referral for additional evaluation if necessary. The nurse can determine if danger signs are present that warrant transportation to an emergency department, or whether the constellation of signs and symptoms warrant the student being picked up by his or her parents and referred to a medical provider for evaluation. The school nurse may also provide parents with written instructions on how

to observe their child for danger signs that may warrant emergency care. When a child who has sustained a concussion returns to school, the school nurse can help with symptom monitoring and provide a place to rest during the school day. He or she may also serve as a resource for other school personnel who have questions about the implications of a student's concussion. This professional can help implement orders from health care professionals and determine if it is appropriate for the student to be in school and whether health-related adjustments need to be continued. The school nurse is essential in collaborating with district administration in the formulation of a concussion management policy. Policies may look quite different from district to district, depending upon the staff and resources available. The nurse can also be a direct liaison to the student's primary health care provider. He or she may obtain the signed release of information allowing for direct communication to clarify orders or reformulate a care plan. The school nurse may then be the team member responsible for informing district staff members about the student's return to activity plan. The school nurse will be particularly involved in cases of students experiencing prolonged recovery or who have sustained multiple concussions. He or she may also help student-athletes understand the relationship between their recovery status and the results of neurocognitive tests that are described later in this book. Finally, the school nurse can help implement prevention and education programs by giving staff, students, and parents information on concussion prevention, identification, and management.

- *Athletic Trainer:* The athletic trainer (AT) can be involved in education and awareness training about concussion at the start of a season. If a child sustains an athletic injury, or sustains a nonathletic injury but expects to continue involvement in school sports, the AT can evaluate possible injuries and make referrals to appropriate care providers. The AT can determine if signs and symptoms of concussion warrant transportation to an emergency department or if parents should be referred to the child's medical provider for evaluation. The AT can also provide parents with written instructions on how to observe the student for complications that may be related to a concussion that indicate emergency care may be warranted. Once a student with a concussion returns to school, the AT can help the school implement the medical provider's recommendations, facilitate communication among all team members, and review the medical provider's recommendations with the student. This professional can help monitor ongoing symptoms and assist with coordinating and supervising the return-to-activity process. He or she can also communicate with the school about the student athlete's ongoing progress. The AT is essential in ensuring that student athletes receive postconcussion care as directed by their medical provider. ATs can also oversee the process of all student athletes taking computerized neurocognitive tests to establish a baseline, retesting after injury, and providing the results to outside medical providers to aid in determining the student's status and degree of recovery. Depending on district policy, the AT may be the designated individual to review and accept the outside medical provider's written clearance to allow a student athlete to return to play. The AT would then inform appropriate district staff of the student's clearance to return to activity.

Athletic team members

- ***Coach:*** Coaches can be involved in the education and awareness training about concussion at the start of a sports season. The coach can help recognize concussion symptoms in players and remove players who may have sustained concussions from athletic play, including practice and competitions. He or she should remove a student who has sustained a significant blow to the head or body and is exhibiting signs or symptoms of concussion from play. Because the coach may not have witnessed the collision, he or she can receive communication from other team members about a student athlete's injury. The coach can contact the school nurse or AT for assistance in evaluating and managing a student's injury. The coach should send students exhibiting any of the danger signs related to head trauma to the nearest hospital emergency department via emergency transport, or follow district policy related to such situations. In less urgent situations, the coach can inform parents of the suspected concussion and refer them to their medical provider, with written information on concussions and the district's concussion management policy. He or she can also communicate with school personnel about the student's injury and subsequent progress upon return to school. The coach should also ensure that a student who was diagnosed with a concussion does not return to participation in athletic activities until he or she has received written clearance from a qualified medical professional.

- **Athletic Director:** The AD is responsible for overseeing the athletic department's concussion team plan. This includes development and management of safety and response policies; education of athletes, coaches, and parents; and equipment management. The AD should be aware of district policies regarding concussion management and act as a liaison between coaches and district staff. The AD will likely be responsible for ensuring that appropriate information is provided to student athletes, parents, and coaches at the outset of each sports season and that the appropriate consent forms are signed for athlete participation. This person can offer additional educational information and programs related to concussions and sports safety. The AD must inform the school nurse, the AT, and the CTL of any student suspected of having a concussion. He or she can then ensure that the student is not permitted to participate in athletic activity, practice, or play until they secure a written clearance from a qualified medical professional is received. The AD is also responsible for making sure coaches know and understand district protocols related to emergency medical transport of students who are injured during interscholastic athletic events, including practice. The athletic director (AD) is advised to keep yearly logs of concussed athletes who play multiple sports. Finally, the AD must enforce district concussion policies, including training of athletic personnel and return to play protocols.
- **PE Teacher:** The PE teacher can help ensure that students are following recommended guidelines for physical activity following concussion. The PE teacher can also find alternative ways for such students to be involved in the lessons or activities. He or she can assist with observing a student's symptoms and recovery trajectory. This professional would report any students with observed signs or reported symptoms to the CTL.

THE CTL

The CTL or case manager will serve as the primary point of contact for all team members, including the student and his or her parents/guardians. This person will be the primary advocate for the student's needs. He or she will also convene team meetings, ensure adequate communication among team members, and facilitate a seamless implementation of an accommodation plan. Other responsibilities will likely include overseeing the return-to-learn process and getting a release of information (ROI) document in order to speak with the student's physician about medical care and the improvement trajectory.

Every school and district is different; therefore, there is flexibility in overall team membership and in who might be appointed as the CTL. Depending upon the roles and responsibilities of different professionals in the school, the CTL might be the school psychologist, school nurse, school counselor, an administrator, or someone else. The designated individual should be organized, have excellent communication and collaboration skills, understand the importance of data-based decision making and progress monitoring, be willing to learn, and be in the school building most days. In many cases, the logical choice is the person who serves as the building's Section 504 or Intervention Assistance Team Coordinator, as many of the same skills can transfer to the CTL role.

At the onset of the school year, the CTL should be made known to everyone within the school community, including parents, teachers, coaches, and athletes. This lets everyone know to whom concussive injuries should be reported. Depending upon the size of the district and the extent of support staff available, the school concussion team may elect to have two leaders: the CTL, who would also serve as the academic leader (AL) or medical leader (ML), as well as a second individual who would take the lead role in academic or medical concussion management (Nationwide Children's Hospital, 2012b).

Exhibit 3.1 shows three sample high schools that have concussion teams comprised of different professionals. The team members listed for each school are consistent members across the school year. The student, parent(s), and physician obviously change for each case.

In the first example in Exhibit 3.1, if Kennedy High School's CTL is the school nurse, that person would also serve as the ML, and the designated AL is someone from the "academic team"—in this case, the school counselor. However, at Jefferson High School the CTL is the school psychologist, who also serves as the AL. In this school, the second leader is someone from the medical team; the nurse's aide serves as the ML.

In schools that do not have sufficient resources to split the medical and academic duties, the CTL may be responsible for both the medical and academic assessments and accommodation coordination. This is generally the school nurse, school psychologist, school counselor, or an

EXHIBIT 3.1

Sample Concussion Team Structures With One Versus Two Leaders

TWO-LEADER MODELS		ONE-LEADER MODEL
KENNEDY HIGH SCHOOL	**JEFFERSON HIGH SCHOOL**	**WASHINGTON HIGH SCHOOL**
CTL/ML: School nurse	*CTL/AL:* School psychologist	*CTL:* School administrator
AL: Lead school counselor	*ML:* Nurse's aide	
Members: Principal, AD, athletic trainer, all other school counselors (one per grade level)	*Members:* Assistant principal, speech-language pathologist, lead PE teacher, AD	*Members:* School counselor, district nurse, head football coach

AD, athletic director; CTL, concussion team leader; ML, medical leaders; PE, physical education.

administrator. For example, Washington High School is a smaller, rural school with few support services. While related service personnel are members of the concussion team, the school has only one designated leader.

CONCUSSION MANAGEMENT PROCESS

A number of models describe a process of concussion management within a team framework. This can be individualized to meet school and district needs. In general, the first step is to inform the school community that there is a specific process to be followed for each school. This information should be shared with district personnel, students, and families. Following is some simple, suggested language that can be modified based on district need. This type of memo can be shared in school newsletters, as e-mail blasts, or on district websites:

> *Dear Staff and Parents:*
>
> [**Insert name of school**] is implementing a concussion team model to help students who have sustained concussions safely return to school. Team members include: [**insert names of concussion team members and their professional roles within the school**].

(continued)

> If you know or suspect your child has sustained a concussion, please contact **[insert concussion team leader's name and contact information]** right away. The team can then develop a plan of academic adjustments to help your child when he or she returns to school.
>
> Sincerely,
>
> **[insert name and title of school principal and/or concussion team leader]**

Then, once a concussion case is confirmed and the team has met with the family to devise an academic accommodation plan, a more extensive letter can be distributed to the student's teachers. It might read something like this:

> *Dear* **[staff member name or role]**,
>
> **[Insert student name]** sustained a concussion on **[date]**. We ask that you assist with **[his/her]** concussion management and recovery.
>
> Each concussion can cause different symptoms. Some symptoms may appear right away and some may develop over time. Some students recovering from a concussion may need to stay home from school to rest for a few days before returning to school. Most students who have sustained concussions will be better within a few weeks, but some can take months to recover. Many return to school while they still have some symptoms and managing these symptoms appropriately can help with recovery. Common signs and symptoms of concussion include:
>
> | Signs (observed by others) | Symptoms (reported by the student) |
> |---|---|
> | | **Cognitive (thinking)** |
> | • Appears dazed or confused | • Feeling slowed down |
> | • Is confused about events | • Difficulty concentrating |
> | • Answers questions slowly | • Difficulty remembering new information |
> | • Repeats questions | |
> | • Can't recall events prior to and/or after the hit, bump, or fall | **Physical** |
> | | • Headache |
> | • Loses consciousness (even briefly) | • Fuzzy or blurry vision |

(continued)

• Shows behavior or personality changes • Forgets class schedule or assignments	• Nausea or vomiting (early on) • Sensitivity to noise or light • Balance problems • Feeling tired/having no energy **Emotional/Mood** • Irritability • Sadness • More emotional • Nervousness or anxiety **Sleep** • Sleeping more than usual • Sleeping less than usual • Trouble falling asleep

A student who has sustained a concussion needs to rest the brain following injury. This includes avoiding bright lights and loud noises (including dances, sporting events, TV, loud music, video games, smartboards, and computers). Cognitive activities such as reading and problem solving may need to be adjusted.

Attached is an **Academic Adjustment Plan** that indicates school-based adjustments selected by the concussion team and/or the student's physician for optimal healing based on this student's symptoms. Please be flexible and understand healing takes place at different rates. Please contact **[concussion team leader name and contact info]** if you have any questions or to report any worsening of symptoms.

Thank you.

[name and role]

Concussion Team Leader

Source: Adapted from ORCAS' Brain 101: The Concussion Playbook.

The following concussion team process (Exhibit 3.2) is adapted from *Nationwide Children's Hospital's Concussion Toolkit* (Nationwide Children's Hospital, 2012b). A key benefit of the process is that it is flexible, allowing it to meet the needs of districts of different sizes with varying demographics.

3. THE CONCUSSION TEAM MODEL   55

Step 1
- School community informed about reporting process
- Concussion reported to concussion team leader

Step 2
- Contact student and family
- Meet with student upon return to school

Step 3
- Assess medical needs
- Use medical documentation if available

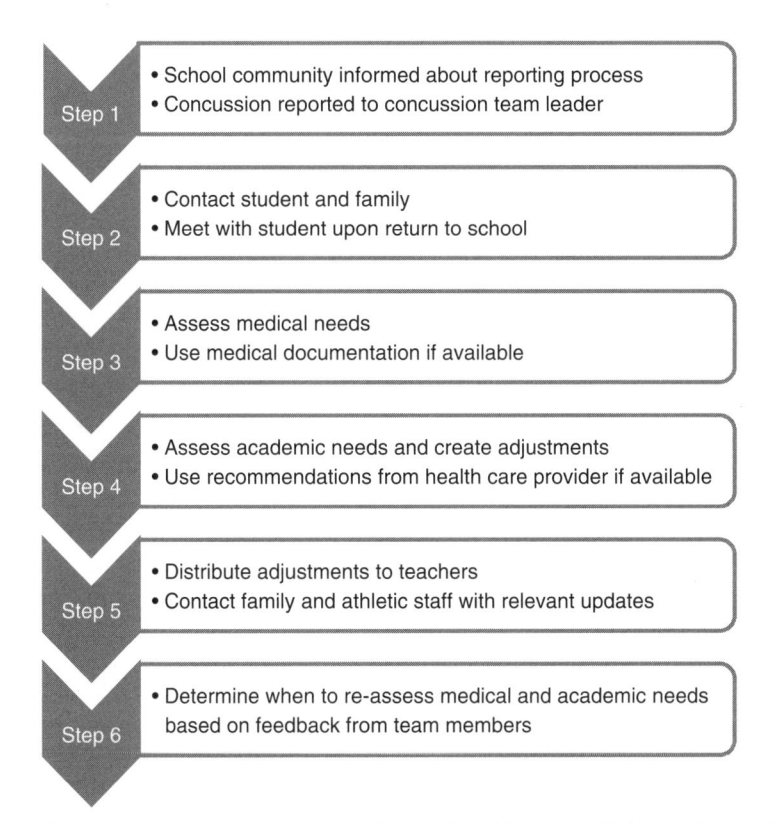

Step 4
- Assess academic needs and create adjustments
- Use recommendations from health care provider if available

Step 5
- Distribute adjustments to teachers
- Contact family and athletic staff with relevant updates

Step 6
- Determine when to re-assess medical and academic needs based on feedback from team members

Figure 3.2. Concussion team process. Adapted from Nationwide Children's Hospital. (2012a).

1. **Step 1. Concussion reported.** Step 1 allows for the possibility that a concussion may be reported to anyone within the school setting. A parent might call the school nurse. A student might alert the teacher. A coach might tell the AD. Any concussions reported to anyone within the school setting are to be reported to the CTL as soon as possible.

2. **Step 2. Contact student and family.** The CTL and/or the concussion team will meet with the student upon his or her return to school, even if the return involves a partial day. For younger students, this initial meeting will also involve the parents. For older students, parents can be included, but this is not required to carry out the remaining steps. The CTL will explain his or role, provide contact information, and describe next steps in the process. The CTL will also describe what is expected from the student and family, including honest communication, adhering to recommendations, and the two-way sharing (with a signed release)

of information and documentation with the physician. This initial contact is essential for ensuring good communication with—and compliance from—the student and his or her family.

3. **Step 3. Assess medical needs.** This step involves gathering documentation, if available, from a physician and/or AT. This documentation may specify recommendations concerning restrictions from cognitive and physical activity, as well as recommended adjustments to the learning environment. Sometimes, a school team knows that a student has sustained a concussion, but no specific recommendations are available from a medical provider. In such cases, the CTL or designated ML, such as the school nurse, should conduct a symptom assessment to determine whether the concussed student will benefit from being at school, whether there should be a modified school day, or whether any attendance at school is likely to be counterproductive. The *Concussion Symptom Tracking Log* (see Chapter 4) can assist with this assessment. Students whose symptoms are severe will likely need to be sent home. However, if symptoms are mild and manageable, and are not exacerbated by being at school, the process can continue to Step 4.

4. **Step 4. Assess academic needs.** Once a student is back to school for partial or full days, the school team can begin to implement any necessary and appropriate academic adjustments. The medical provider may send the parents or the school recommendations for academic adjustments. Such recommendations should be incorporated into a specific, written plan. If no recommendations are available, or if the recommendations are vague or no longer relevant (due to rapid healing that can take place after a concussion), the CTL or designated AL should assess the concussed student's academic needs. The *Classroom Concussion Assessment Form* and other information found in the next chapter can assist with this process.

5. **Step 5. Distribute adjustments.** The plan for adjusting the learning environment and academic expectations is then distributed in writing to the student's teachers, family, and (if applicable) athletic staff by the CTL. Updates to medical information are included as well. Chapter 6 contains detailed information on how to map the assessed academic needs onto appropriate school-based adjustments.

6. **Step 6. Determine reassessment.** The CTL will identify an appropriate timeline for reassessment of needs to ensure that adjustments are not maintained for an unnecessary length of time. This can also help team members determine if new adjustments

may be required to address new symptoms or issues. This is determined based on data and feedback from the team; the team should go back to Steps 3 or 4 as needed. It is recommended that the team reassess medical and/or academic needs when:

- New physician documentation arrives dictating a new course of action
- Symptoms have changed (and therefore the prior assessment needs to be altered)
- Symptoms have resolved and are no longer a barrier to school participation or attendance
- Teachers or parents identify problems in the current plan that are not being adequately addressed

Once the reassessment is complete, the CTL will document the results and return to Step 5, notify relevant parties of any changes to the plan, then continue to Step 6, identify appropriate time frame for reassessment (Nationwide Children's Hospital, 2012b).

Ben

While Ben's recreational league football coaches and parents could have used more education about concussion causes, signs, and symptoms prior to the start of his football season, his elementary school's concussion team had a coordinated and proactive response.

Ben's mother took him to the emergency department the night after he sustained a significant blow to the body during his football game. He was diagnosed with a concussion and received general recommendations upon discharge, including that he "avoid physical activity and reduce cognitive demands (reading, texting, computer use, video games, etc.)." The doctor indicated that school attendance and after-school activity may need to be modified to avoid increasing symptoms. The written discharge instructions also suggested that Ben's parents contact his physician or another physician who was knowledgeable about concussion management after leaving the emergency department. While these are good general recommendations, Ben's parents decided that he didn't need to see another doctor and they would just let him rest.

Ben stayed at home from school for 2 days, mostly watching television and listening to music with his headphones. Because those activities were not specified as off-limits on the emergency department discharge form, his mother thought it would be fine. After the second day, Ben's mother could not miss any more work and Ben's father was traveling out of town, so Ben went back to school. Ben's mother sent his teacher, Mr. Stevens, an e-mail letting him know that Ben was diagnosed with concussion but now seemed well enough to go back to school.

Ben's school had a concussion management team in place. Mr. Stevens knew the protocol was for him to immediately contact his school's Concussion Team Leader (CTL), Ms. Tippins. Ms. Tippins immediately contacted Ben's mother and asked her to sign a release of information (ROI) to allow her to receive and review Ben's medical evaluation and speak with his doctor. When Ms. Tippins learned that Ben had only been seen in the emergency department, she suggested to Ben's mother that she follow up with a concussion specialist and gave a few recommendations of local physicians. Ms. Tippins emphasized that Ben would benefit from having a qualified medical provider indicate when he could safely return to football practice and play.

"Part of my role is to make sure that Ben's teacher and everyone else here at school understand that Ben has had a concussion and may need a bit of time before he's feeling better." Ms. Tippins told Ben's mom. "I'll be checking in with you over the next few weeks to see how Ben seems at home and to let you know what we're doing at school to make adjustments while Ben's concussion heals. Now, can you tell me how he slept last night?"

Ms. Tippins proceeded to ask Ben's mother specific questions regarding Ben's symptoms using a list of possible symptoms to see if she had observed any of them or if he had complained to her of any. She also asked a few key questions to help the team formulate an appropriate plan of academic adjustments for Ben. She then met with Ben to evaluate which symptoms were present and how intense they were. The outcomes of this assessment and a copy of his academic adjustments can be found in the chapters on concussion assessment (Chapter 4) and Adjustments to the School Environment (Chapter 6).

EDUCATING THE SCHOOL COMMUNITY

Anyone responsible for the student both during and after school hours—including bus drivers and babysitters—should receive information from the concussion team regarding how they can best help the student. They can also help monitor symptoms during recovery by reporting academic, behavioral, or emotional concerns to the CTL.

Educators often deal with situations involving students making excuses for why their schoolwork is not finished. This can lead to some skepticism when someone is asking them to make exceptions for students who have sustained concussions, particularly because this is an invisible injury. Thus, it can be difficult for some teachers to understand if a student is being truthful when he or she continues to complain of symptoms or when a student's parent or doctor reports that a child is taking a long time to heal.

The school-based concussion team can be instrumental in educating the entire school community—teachers, administrators, support personnel, parents, and students themselves—about what a concussion is and what an injured student might be experiencing. Having teachers who are sympathetic and who understand the needs of a concussed student can help provide reassurance to a student that he or she will not fail classes because of missed work or missed days of school. This, in turn, can decrease the student's stress and thus facilitate recovery. By pulling together a team of caring professionals, the CTL can ensure that everyone involved in the student's life—parents or guardians, coaches, teachers, health care providers—is getting the same information and is hearing a consistent message.

More information on training for the school community, including parents and teachers, can be found in Chapter 7.

WORKING WITH PARENTS

It is crucial to involve the family in the transition process; the entire family may be affected by the injury. Parents may become overprotective and restrict previously enjoyed freedoms (e.g., driving to school, bike riding, climbing on playground equipment). This is often extended to siblings.

It is important that school-based members of the concussion team involve parents as equal partners and participants as team members. It is important to listen, validate parents' feelings, avoid defensiveness, recognize fear and frustration, focus on solutions, and work together toward common goals.

Julia

Julia wanted to resume playing soccer while she still had concussion symptoms. She also wanted to push through completing her school assignments so they would not continue looming over her head. In a meeting with the concussion team, Julia's mother was upset.

"This has continued for too long! She's still not better! I just want her on complete bedrest until her symptoms are totally gone."

"There is no way that is happening," muttered Julia.

"Generally, what we see is that students heal the fastest when there is a balance between rest and exertion," explained the athletic trainer. "We'd love to see Julia back on the soccer field, but you're right that she needs more rest from activities before she can be cleared for that. At the same time, most studies have shown that if someone with a concussion just goes into a dark and quiet room without any stimulation, their symptoms actually take longer to get better."

"We want to help Julia find that balance," added the school counselor. "I'm also concerned that Julia has seemed very down since her last concussion." She looked at Julia. "You seem to be pulling away from your friends and social activities. It would be great if we could find some things that you enjoy that don't involve playing sports or being around a very stimulating environment."

"There's nothing," Julia shook her head.

"She wants to be on the move. She always has," Julia's mother said. "She likes loud concerts and mountain climbing and going to the movies—3D with surround sound! There is nothing she really enjoys that doesn't involve a lot of action and noise. But it all makes her symptoms worse, especially the headaches."

"You're absolutely right that those things all might make her concussion symptoms worse and prolong her recovery," validated the school nurse. "But maybe some of those things can be tempered a bit. Like instead of loud concerts, you could listen to acoustic music at a mellow coffee shop."

"Yeah," Julia's concurred. "I like that kind of music, too. But coffee makes my head hurt."

"Try herbal tea," suggested the school nurse.

"Or instead of mountain climbing you could walk in the woods, and instead of loud 3D movies, maybe you could find good movies to watch at a lower volume at home. That way if it makes your symptoms worse at all, you could turn it off and come back to it later," suggested the athletic director.

Julia's mom laughed, "She does seem to like the older movies from the 1980s more than a lot of the newer ones."

"And maybe if you do that, a couple of friends from the soccer team could come over to watch with her," added the school counselor. "Not a big crowd, but just a way to keep that support system going."

"That's a good idea," said Julia's stepfather. "I'll try to get a few of those movies for her."

"And we want the two of you," the school nurse nodded at Julia's mom and stepfather, "and you," she nodded at Julia, "to be sure to tell us if there are any changes in your symptoms, for better or for worse, based on these new adjustments we're putting into place at school. Now, let's go over these possibilities..."

In Julia's case, the team did a nice job of involving both Julia and her parents in a dialogue of problem solving and support. They validated what the "family team" was experiencing and incorporated their input and suggestions, all of which were very important in structuring a plan that made sense for this student.

STUDENT PRIVACY

The benefits of a team approach to concussion management are innumerable. At the same time, any time personnel discuss a student's medical condition and academic performance—particularly when there are electronic communications and multiple forms of data tracking that student's progress—school personnel must be mindful about student privacy.

Health Insurance Portability and Accountability Act

Information about a student's health is protected by the Health Insurance Portability and Accountability Act (HIPPA) of 1996. HIPAA generally applies to protected health information in nonschool settings. Such health information includes that which is related to treatment, assessment, and past, present, or future health conditions. HIPAA requires that medical information not be disclosed to anyone besides the parent or guardian unless otherwise specified in writing. Thus, a signed ROI is important to allow the school to receive and discuss medical information related to a concussion with a student's health care provider. An exception to this is that the HIPAA privacy rule allows health care providers to disclose protected health information about students to school nurses for treatment purposes, without the authorization of the student or the student's parents. This might occur in cases where the school nurse administers students' medication or tends to their other health care needs at school.

Medical providers will likely have their own forms that they also want completed and signed. Such forms generally ask the parent to sign authorization for the health care provider to disclose protected health information to the school. The form may specify that the release of information covers the period of health care for a specific period of time *or* for all past, present, and future periods. The form may also allow the respondent to authorize the release of the student's complete health record or for the complete health record excluding specific exceptions.

Family Educational Rights and Privacy Act

Information on a student's academic record is protected by the Family Educational Rights and Privacy Act (FERPA; 1965b). FERPA protects students' personal information, including that which is related to their name, address, social security number, educational records, and health records obtained by an educational agency that have become part of an educational record. For example, a student's immunization record maintained by an educational agency or the school nurse would be protected by FERPA. Additionally, records maintained by schools related to special education, including records on services provided to students under the Individuals with Disabilities Education Improvement Act (IDEA) of 2004, are considered educational records under FERPA.

All schools that receive funding from the U.S. Department of Education are required to adhere to FERPA regulations. As such, they must secure student educational records against intentional or unintentional release. Under FERPA, parents have the right to inspect and review their child's educational records until their child reaches the age of 18. At that time, the rights transfer to the student. These records cannot be shared with a third party without written parental consent (or the student's consent if he or she is over 18) unless disclosure meets one or more specific exceptions to FERPA's general consent requirement. One such exception allows schools to disclose a student's health and medical information and other educational records to teachers and other school officials, without written consent, if the school officials have "legitimate educational interest" in accordance with school policy. For example, a school counselor who is helping plan a student's next year of classes could review the student's previous coursework without explicit written parental permission.

Another permissible disclosure without explicit written consent is release of records to appropriate parties in connection with an emergency, if knowledge of the information is necessary to protect the health or safety of the student and other individuals (U.S. Department of Health and Human Services and U.S. Department of Education, 2008). For example, there was considerable debate in the academic community following the Virginia Tech shootings about the university's counseling center, campus police, and academic departments all having knowledge about the shooter's violent tendencies. However, each of these departments failed to share critical information about his issues because they believed that doing so violated FERPA. The emergency exception in FERPA may have allowed for sharing among Virginia Tech departments about the shooter's conduct that demonstrated he posed a risk to himself and others, if the threat was imminent (Chapman, 2009).

Staff members should be regularly reminded to only discuss information that is necessary to manage the student's situation. They must also understand how to appropriately communicate what is involved in a student's plan in a way that maintains student privacy. This includes specific directives from the school district regarding electronic communication and the secure storage of student records.

Carly

When Carly was bothered by the bright lights and loud noises the day after falling from the monkey bars, Carly's teacher, Mrs. Lang, went into the office. After a parent volunteer who was making copies left the room, Mrs. Lang asked the attendance secretary for more information about Carly's fall and subsequent behavior in the office the day before.

The nurse was in the office that day, so Mrs. Lang relayed the situation to her. The nurse then pulled Carly's health form to see if there were any reports of a previous history of concussions and asked Mrs. Lang to send Carly down to see her.

While the school's failure to inform Carly's parents about her fall from the monkey bars the day of the injury was a significant misstep, they handled communication about the incident the next day appropriately. Because the secretary had seen Carly immediately after the injury and the nurse was knowledgeable about concussions, it was appropriate for both of them to discuss this situation with Carly's teacher. People were involved on a "need to know" basis. Mrs. Lang did not discuss Carly's accident in front of a parent volunteer and the school nurse accessed a medical record that was part of a school record because there was a legitimate educational interest.

The U.S. Department of Education and the U.S. Department of Health and Human Services published a joint guidance document on the application of FERPA and HIPPA of 1996 to student records (www2.ed.gov/policy/gen/guid/fpco/doc/ferpa-hippa-guidance.pdf), which can provide information to school teams on their rights and restrictions in terms of accessing and sharing student information.

SUSTAINABILITY OF THE MODEL

A *written procedure* needs to outline a coordinated communication plan among appropriate staff to not only ensure that postconcussion management plans are implemented and followed for individual students, but also that the team model is sustained from year to year. It is important that school personnel make sure that the protocol is not depending upon a specific person or role. It is also essential that the concussion team model include a procedure for periodic review of the team structure and the concussion management policy, given the changes in concussion protocol that grow out of research.

REFERENCES

Chapman, K. (2009). A preventable tragedy at Virginia Tech: Why confusion over FERPA's provisions prevent schools from addressing student violence. *Public Interest Law Journal, 18*, 349–385.

Family Educational Rights and Privacy Act, as amended. Codified at 20 U.S.C. § 1232g (1965a).

Family Educational Rights and Privacy Act Regulations. 34 C.F.R. Part 99 (1965b). http://www2.ed.gov/policy/gen/guid/fpco/ferpa/index.html

Halstead, M. E., McAvoy, K., Devord, C., Carl, R., Lee, M., Logan, K., ... Council on School Health. (2013). Returning to learning following a concussion. *American Academy of Pediatrics, 132*(5), 948–957. doi:10.1542/Peds.2013-2867

Health Insurance Portability and Accountability Act of 1996, as amended. Codified at 42 U.S.C. § 1320d et seq. and § 300gg; and 29 U.S.C. § 1181 et seq. P.L. No. 104–191, 110 Stat. 1938 (1996).

Individuals with Disabilities Education Improvement Act, 20 U.S.C. § 1400 (2004).

McAvoy, K. (2011). *REAP the benefits of good concussion management.* Centennial, CO: Rocky Mountain Sports Medicine Institute Center for Concussion. Retrieved from: http://rockymountainhospitalforchildren.com/service/concussion-management-reap-guidelines

Nationwide Children's Hospital. (2012a). *A school administrator's guide to academic concussion management.* Retrieved from http://www.nationwidechildrens.org/concussions-in-the-classroom

Nationwide Children's Hospital. (2012b). *Concussion toolkit.* Retrieved from http://www.nationwidechildrens.org/concussion-toolkit

ORCAS. (2013). Staff notification letter. *Brain 101: The concussion playbook.* Retrieved from: http://orcas-sportsconc2.s3.amazonaws.com/files/h_staff_letter.pdf

Sady, M. D., Vaughan, C. G., & Gioia, G. A. (2011). School and the concussed youth: Recommendations for concussion education and management. *Physical Medicine and Rehabilitation Clinics of North America, 22*(4), 701–719. doi:10.1016/j.pmr.2011.08.008

U.S. Department of Health and Human Services and U.S. Department of Education. (2008). Joint Guidance on the Application of the Family Education Rights and Privacy Act (FERPA) and the Health Insurance Portability and Accountability Act of 1996 (HIPAA) to Student Health Records. Retrieved from www2.ed.gov/policy/gen/guid/fpco/doc/ferpa-hippa-guidance.pdf

CHAPTER 4

Concussion Assessment

While the diagnosis of a concussion needs to be made by a medical professional, a concussion is both a medical and an educational issue. Concussions may occur in an educational setting and therefore school personnel may serve as first responders. Further, this medical issue can lead to educational needs that must be addressed with school-based accommodations. School personnel need to be informed about concussion assessments that occur in the medical and athletic setting. They also need assessment tools to track a student's recovery and evaluate the efficacy of academic adjustments.

In this chapter, the reader first learns about simple tools that can be used by school personnel to assess concussion symptomology at school. These include checklists that can be used by nurses or other school staff when a concussion is sustained at school. There is also information on the use of computerized neurocognitive assessments and sideline assessments for student athletes. Additionally, smartphone concussion evaluation apps are discussed and guidelines for appropriate use are described. The chapter also includes information related to the clinical evaluation of a concussion that a child might receive in a medical setting.

Next is information on how school personnel can conduct ongoing assessment of a student's concussion symptoms, as well as progress monitoring of the efficacy of academic adjustments. The chapter concludes with a brief section on the future of concussion assessment. Readers are advised to stay current on this information, as medical and technological advances may soon lead to more sensitive tests that allow for more objective evaluations of concussions.

CONCUSSION SIGNS AND SYMPTOMS CHECKLISTS

Children and adolescents who have sustained a concussion will experience one or more symptoms from one or more of the symptom categories described in Chapter 2 (physical, cognitive, emotional, and sleep). The *Concussion Signs and Symptoms Checklist* (see Exhibit 4.1), provided free of charge from the Centers for Disease Control and Prevention (CDC), can be used to monitor observed signs (physical, cognitive, emotional) if a student sustains a possible concussion at school, or if the student arrives at school reporting a possible head injury that occurred earlier, outside of school or on a previous school day. It is recommended that the concussion team leader (CTL) and main office staff keep copies of these checklists on hand for use in the case of any suspected concussion.

The evaluator uses the form to check for signs or symptoms upon arrival, 15 minutes later, at the end of 30 minutes, and before the student leaves. Children experiencing one or more signs should be referred to a health care professional with experience in evaluating concussions. The evaluator should provide a copy of the form to the parents to give to the doctor and keep a copy for school records.

In addition to listing possible signs of a concussion, the form has a section on *Danger Signs*, which indicate the student should be seen in the emergency department right away. The form also includes a section for documenting resolution of injury and comments. The name and title of the person completing the form are also included, which allows an outside medical professional to know the background of the person completing the form, be it the school nurse, an office aide, or someone else.

Carly

When Carly returned to school she told Mrs. Lang that she had a headache and felt "funny." Mrs. Lang sent Carly down to the nurse's office. The nurse completed the CDC's Concussion Signs and Symptoms Checklist (Exhibit 4.2) based on how Carly appeared and what she was reporting at that time.

While it would have been better if this checklist had been completed upon injury, this documentation allowed the school staff to make a more informed decision about what to do next. They called her mother and recommended that she take Carly to the doctor to be evaluated for a concussion. They asked her to take a copy of the Signs and Symptoms Checklist with her and made a copy for their records.

EXHIBIT 4.1

Concussion Signs and Symptoms Checklist.

Concussion Signs and Symptoms
Checklist

HEADS UP SCHOOLS

KNOW YOUR CONCUSSION ABCs
Assess the situation | Be alert for signs and symptoms | Contact a health care professional

Student's Name: _____ Student's Grade: _____ Date/Time of Injury: _____

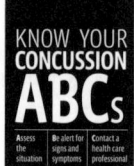

Where and How Injury Occurred: *(Be sure to include cause and force of the hit or blow to the head.)* _____

Description of Injury: *(Be sure to include information about any loss of consciousness and for how long, memory loss, or seizures following the injury, or previous concussions, if any. See the section on Danger Signs on the back of this form.)* _____

DIRECTIONS:

Use this checklist to monitor students who come to your office with a head injury. Students should be monitored for a minimum of 30 minutes. Check for signs or symptoms when the student first arrives at your office, fifteen minutes later, and at the end of 30 minutes.

Students who experience *one or more* of the signs or symptoms of concussion after a bump, blow, or jolt to the head should be referred to a health care professional with experience in evaluating for concussion. For those instances when a parent is coming to take the student to a health care professional, observe the student for any new or worsening symptoms right before the student leaves. Send a copy of this checklist with the student for the health care professional to review.

To download this checklist in Spanish, please visit: www.cdc.gov/Concussion.
Para obtener una copia electrónica de esta lista de síntomas en español, por favor visite: www.cdc.gov/Concussion.

OBSERVED SIGNS	0 MINUTES	15 MINUTES	30 MINUTES	MINUTES Just prior to leaving
Appears dazed or stunned				
Is confused about events				
Repeats questions				
Answers questions slowly				
Can't recall events *prior* to the hit, bump, or fall				
Can't recall events *after* the hit, bump, or fall				
Loses consciousness (even briefly)				
Shows behavior or personality changes				
Forgets class schedule or assignments				
PHYSICAL SYMPTOMS				
Headache or "pressure" in head				
Nausea or vomiting				
Balance problems or dizziness				
Fatigue or feeling tired				
Blurry or double vision				
Sensitivity to light				
Sensitivity to noise				
Numbness or tingling				
Does not "feel right"				
COGNITIVE SYMPTOMS				
Difficulty thinking clearly				
Difficulty concentrating				
Difficulty remembering				
Feeling more slowed down				
Feeling sluggish, hazy, foggy, or groggy				
EMOTIONAL SYMPTOMS				
Irritable				
Sad				
More emotional than usual				
Nervous				

4. CONCUSSION ASSESSMENT

Danger Signs:

Be alert for symptoms that worsen over time. The student should be seen in an emergency department right away if s/he has:

- ❏ One pupil (the black part in the middle of the eye) larger than the other
- ❏ Drowsiness or cannot be awakened
- ❏ A headache that gets worse and does not go away
- ❏ Weakness, numbness, or decreased coordination
- ❏ Repeated vomiting or nausea
- ❏ Slurred speech
- ❏ Convulsions or seizures
- ❏ Difficulty recognizing people or places
- ❏ Increasing confusion, restlessness, or agitation
- ❏ Unusual behavior
- ❏ Loss of consciousness (even a brief loss of consciousness should be taken seriously)

Additional Information About This Checklist:

This checklist is also useful if a student appears to have sustained a head injury outside of school or on a previous school day. In such cases, be sure to ask the student about possible sleep symptoms. Drowsiness, sleeping more or less than usual, or difficulty falling asleep may indicate a concussion.

To maintain confidentiality and ensure privacy, this checklist is intended only for use by appropriate school professionals, health care professionals, and the student's parent(s) or guardian(s).

For a free tear-off pad with additional copies of this form, or for more information on concussion, visit: www.cdc.gov/Concussion.

Resolution of Injury:

__ Student returned to class
__ Student sent home
__ Student referred to health care professional with experience in evaluating for concussion

---

SIGNATURE OF SCHOOL PROFESSIONAL COMPLETING THIS FORM: _____

TITLE: _____

COMMENTS:

For more information on concussion and to order additional materials for school professionals **FREE-OF-CHARGE**, visit: www.cdc.gov/Concussion.

U.S. DEPARTMENT OF HEALTH AND HUMAN SERVICES
CENTERS FOR DISEASE CONTROL AND PREVENTION

From Centers for Disease Control and Prevention.

The "takeaway" from this scenario is that the nurse does not have to be the one to complete the Signs and Symptoms Checklist. This tool, or a similar one, should be readily available to anyone in the school who might be informed about a student's possible concussion, including all office staff. It is not used to make a definitive medical diagnosis, but it can be a valuable piece of information to give to the parents, who can then share it with the medical provider. There is a line on the form for the "title" of the person completing the form, so any medical provider reviewing the form would know if was completed by a nonmedical informant.

EXHIBIT 4.2

Carly's concussion signs and symptoms checklist.

Concussion Signs and Symptoms
Checklist

HEADS UP SCHOOLS — **KNOW YOUR CONCUSSION ABCs**: Assess the situation | Be alert for signs and symptoms | Contact a health care professional

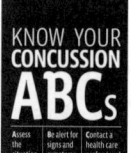

Student's Name: Carly Sutton **Student's Grade:** 1 **Date/Time of Injury:** 3/4/xx 12:45 pm

Where and How Injury Occurred: *(Be sure to include cause and force of the hit or blow to the head.)* Carly fell head first from the monkey bars yesterday (3/4), per report from Carly and a classmate.

Description of Injury: *(Be sure to include information about any loss of consciousness and for how long, memory loss, or seizures following the injury, or previous concussions, if any. See the section on Danger Signs on the back of this form.)* No loss of consciousness, memory loss or danger signs observed

DIRECTIONS:

Use this checklist to monitor students who come to your office with a head injury. Students should be monitored for a minimum of 30 minutes. Check for signs or symptoms when the student first arrives at your office, fifteen minutes later, and at the end of 30 minutes.

Students who experience *one or more* of the signs or symptoms of concussion after a bump, blow, or jolt to the head should be referred to a health care professional with experience in evaluating for concussion. For those instances when a parent is coming to take the student to a health care professional, observe the student for any new or worsening symptoms right before the student leaves. Send a copy of this checklist with the student for the health care professional to review.

To download this checklist in Spanish, please visit: www.cdc.gov/Concussion. Para obtener una copia electrónica de esta lista de síntomas en español, por favor visite: www.cdc.gov/Concussion.

May 2010

OBSERVED SIGNS	0 MINUTES	15 MINUTES	30 MINUTES	37 MINUTES *Just prior to leaving*
Appears dazed or stunned				
Is confused about events				
Repeats questions				
Answers questions slowly				
Can't recall events *prior* to the hit, bump, or fall				
Can't recall events *after* the hit, bump, or fall				
Loses consciousness (even briefly)				
Shows behavior or personality changes	✓	✓	✓	✓
Forgets class schedule or assignments				
PHYSICAL SYMPTOMS				
Headache or "pressure" in head	✓	✓	✓	✓
Nausea or vomiting				
Balance problems or dizziness				
Fatigue or feeling tired	✓	✓	✓	✓
Blurry or double vision				
Sensitivity to light	✓	✓	✓	✓
Sensitivity to noise	✓	✓	✓	✓
Numbness or tingling				
Does not "feel right"	✓	✓	✓	✓
COGNITIVE SYMPTOMS				
Difficulty thinking clearly				
Difficulty concentrating				
Difficulty remembering				
Feeling more slowed down				
Feeling sluggish, hazy, foggy, or groggy	✓	✓	✓	✓
EMOTIONAL SYMPTOMS				
Irritable				
Sad				
More emotional than usual	✓	✓	✓	✓
Nervous				

→ More

Danger Signs:

Be alert for symptoms that worsen over time. The student should be seen in an emergency department right away if s/he has:

- ❏ One pupil (the black part in the middle of the eye) larger than the other
- ❏ Drowsiness or cannot be awakened
- ❏ A headache that gets worse and does not go away
- ❏ Weakness, numbness, or decreased coordination
- ❏ Repeated vomiting or nausea
- ❏ Slurred speech
- ❏ Convulsions or seizures
- ❏ Difficulty recognizing people or places
- ❏ Increasing confusion, restlessness, or agitation
- ❏ Unusual behavior
- ❏ Loss of consciousness (even a brief loss of consciousness should be taken seriously)

Additional Information About This Checklist:

This checklist is also useful if a student appears to have sustained a head injury outside of school or on a previous school day. In such cases, be sure to ask the student about possible sleep symptoms. Drowsiness, sleeping more or less than usual, or difficulty falling asleep may indicate a concussion.

To maintain confidentiality and ensure privacy, this checklist is intended only for use by appropriate school professionals, health care professionals, and the student's parent(s) or guardian(s).

For a free tear-off pad with additional copies of this form, or for more information on concussion, visit: www.cdc.gov/Concussion.

Resolution of Injury:

___ Student returned to class
X Student sent home
___ Student referred to health care professional with experience in evaluating for concussion

SIGNATURE OF SCHOOL PROFESSIONAL COMPLETING THIS FORM: _____

TITLE: School Nurse

COMMENTS:
After yesterday's fall, Carly appeared fine to the playground aide and she was sent back to class. Today she came to my office exhibiting several signs and symptoms consistent with concussion.
I monitored her in my office until her mother could pick her up from school. Carly is typically very bubbly and talkative. She was quiet and seemed "off" and spacy — not like herself.

For more information on concussion and to order additional materials for school professionals FREE-OF-CHARGE, visit: www.cdc.gov/Concussion.

U.S. DEPARTMENT OF HEALTH AND HUMAN SERVICES
CENTERS FOR DISEASE CONTROL AND PREVENTION

Another useful form from the CDC is the *Acute Concussion Evaluation* (ACE; Gioia & Collins, 2006) for initial evaluations (see Figure 4.1). The ACE can help the school concussion team obtain information regarding the injury, including the cause, severity, any amnesia, loss of consciousness, and any early signs. The form asks the patient to report the presence of symptoms in four categories:

thinking/remembering, physical, emotional, sleep. It also assesses for risk factors, such as history of injury, developmental history, and psychiatric history; provides a warning of red-flags and applicable diagnostic codes; and encourages the development of a follow-up

---

ACUTE CONCUSSION EVALUATION (ACE)
PHYSICIAN/CLINICIAN OFFICE VERSION
Gerard Gioia, PhD[1] & Micky Collins, PhD[2]
[1]Children's National Medical Center
[2]University of Pittsburgh Medical Center

Patient Name:_____
DOB: _____ Age:_____
Date:_____ ID/MR#_____

A. Injury Characteristics   Date/Time of Injury_____   Reporter: __Patient __Parent __Spouse __Other_____

1. Injury Description _____

1a. Is there evidence of a forcible blow to the head (direct or indirect)?   __Yes __No __Unknown
1b. Is there evidence of intracranial injury or skull fracture?   __Yes __No __Unknown
1c. Location of Impact: __Frontal __Lft Temporal __Rt Temporal __Lft Parietal __Rt Parietal __Occipital __Neck __Indirect Force
2. Cause: __MVC __Pedestrian-MVC __Fall __Assault __Sports (specify)_____ Other_____
3. Amnesia Before (Retrograde) Are there any events just BEFORE the injury that you/ person has no memory of (even brief)?   __Yes __No Duration____
4. Amnesia After (Anterograde) Are there any events just AFTER the injury that you/ person has no memory of (even brief)?   __Yes __No Duration____
5. Loss of Consciousness: Did you/ person lose consciousness?   __Yes __No Duration____
6. EARLY SIGNS: __Appears dazed or stunned   __Is confused about events   __Answers questions slowly   __Repeats Questions   __Forgetful (recent info)
7. Seizures: Were seizures observed? No__ Yes___ Detail_____

B. Symptom Check List* Since the injury, has the person experienced <u>any</u> of these symptoms any <u>more than usual</u> today or in the past day?
Indicate presence of each symptom (0=No, 1=Yes).   *Lovell & Collins, 1998 JHTR

PHYSICAL (10)			COGNITIVE (4)			SLEEP (4)		
Headache	0	1	Feeling mentally foggy	0	1	Drowsiness	0	1
Nausea	0	1	Feeling slowed down	0	1	Sleeping less than usual	0	1 N/A
Vomiting	0	1	Difficulty concentrating	0	1	Sleeping more than usual	0	1 N/A
Balance problems	0	1	Difficulty remembering	0	1	Trouble falling asleep	0	1 N/A
Dizziness	0	1	COGNITIVE Total (0-4) ____			SLEEP Total (0-4) ____		
Visual problems	0	1	EMOTIONAL (4)					
Fatigue	0	1	Irritability	0	1	**Exertion:** Do these symptoms <u>worsen</u> with:		
Sensitivity to light	0	1	Sadness	0	1	Physical Activity __Yes __No __N/A		
Sensitivity to noise	0	1	More emotional	0	1	Cognitive Activity __Yes __No __N/A		
Numbness/Tingling	0	1	Nervousness	0	1	**Overall Rating:** How <u>different</u> is the person acting compared to his/her usual self? (circle)		
PHYSICAL Total (0-10) ____			EMOTIONAL Total (0-4) ____			Normal 0 1 2 3 4 5 6 Very Different		
(Add Physical, Cognitive, Emotion, Sleep totals) Total Symptom Score (0-22) ____								

C. Risk Factors for Protracted Recovery (check all that apply)

Concussion History? Y ___ N___	√	Headache History? Y ___ N___	√	Developmental History	√	Psychiatric History
Previous # 1 2 3 4 5 6+		Prior treatment for headache		Learning disabilities		Anxiety
Longest symptom duration Days__ Weeks__ Months__ Years__		History of migraine headache __ Personal __ Family_____		Attention-Deficit/ Hyperactivity Disorder		Depression
						Sleep disorder
If multiple concussions, less force caused reinjury? Yes__ No__				Other developmental disorder_____		Other psychiatric disorder _____

List other comorbid medical disorders or medication usage (e.g., hypothyroid, seizures)_____

D. RED FLAGS for acute emergency management: Refer to the emergency department with <u>sudden onset</u> of any of the following:
* Headaches that worsen   * Looks very drowsy/ can't be awakened   * Can't recognize people or places   * Neck pain
* Seizures   * Repeated vomiting   * Increasing confusion or irritability * Unusual behavioral change
* Focal neurologic signs   * Slurred speech   * Weakness or numbness in arms/legs   * Change in state of consciousness

E. Diagnosis (ICD): __Concussion w/o LOC 850.0 __Concussion w/ LOC 850.1 __Concussion (Unspecified) 850.9 __Other (854)_____
                       __No diagnosis

F. Follow-Up Action Plan   Complete *ACE Care Plan* and provide copy to patient/family.
___ No Follow-Up Needed
___ Physician/Clinician Office Monitoring: Date of next follow-up _____
___ Referral:
    ___ Neuropsychological Testing
    ___ Physician: Neurosurgery____ Neurology____ Sports Medicine____ Physiatrist____ Psychiatrist____ Other_____
    ___ Emergency Department

ACE Completed by:_____   © Copyright G. Gioia & M. Collins, 2006

This form is part of the "Heads Up: Brain Injury in Your Practice" tool kit developed by the Centers for Disease Control and Prevention (CDC).

4. CONCUSSION ASSESSMENT

A concussion (or mild traumatic brain injury (MTBI)) is a complex pathophysiologic process affecting the brain, induced by traumatic biomechanical forces secondary to direct or indirect forces to the head. Disturbance of brain function is related to neurometabolic dysfunction, rather than structural injury, and is typically associated with normal structural neuroimaging findings (i.e., CT scan, MRI). Concussion may or may not involve a loss of consciousness (LOC). Concussion results in a constellation of physical, cognitive, emotional, and sleep-related symptoms. Symptoms may last from several minutes to days, weeks, months or even longer in some cases.

ACE Instructions
The ACE is intended to provide an evidence-based clinical protocol to conduct an initial evaluation and diagnosis of patients (both children and adults) with known or suspected MTBI. The research evidence documenting the importance of these components in the evaluation of an MTBI is provided in the reference list.

A. Injury Characteristics:
1. Obtain **description of the injury** – how injury occurred, type of force, location on the head or body (if force transmitted to head). Different biomechanics of injury may result in differential symptom patterns (e.g., occipital blow may result in visual changes, balance difficulties).
2. Indicate the **cause of injury**. Greater forces associated with the trauma are likely to result in more severe presentation of symptoms.
3/4. **Amnesia:** Amnesia is defined as the failure to form new memories. Determine whether amnesia has occurred and attempt to determine length of time of memory dysfunction – **before** (retrograde) and **after** (anterograde) injury. Even seconds to minutes of memory loss can be predictive of outcome. Recent research has indicated that amnesia may be up to 4-10 times more predictive of symptoms and cognitive deficits following concussion than is LOC (less than 1 minute).[1]
5. **Loss of consciousness (LOC)** – If occurs, determine length of LOC.
6. **Early signs.** If present, ask the individuals who know the patient (parent, spouse, friend, etc) about specific signs of the concussion that may have been observed. These signs are typically observed early after the injury.
7. Inquire whether **seizures** were observed or not.

B. Symptom Checklist:[2]
1. Ask patient (and/or parent, if child) to report presence of the four categories of symptoms since injury. It is important to assess all listed symptoms as different parts of the brain control different functions. One or all symptoms may be present depending upon mechanisms of injury.[3] Record "1" for Yes or "0" for No for their presence or absence, respectively.
2. For all symptoms, indicate presence of symptoms as experienced within the past 24 hours. Since symptoms can be present premorbidly/at baseline (e.g., inattention, headaches, sleep, sadness), it is important to assess change from their usual presentation.
3. **Scoring:** Sum total number of symptoms present per area, and sum all four areas into Total Symptom Score (score range 0-22). (Note: most sleep symptoms are only applicable after a night has passed since the injury. Drowsiness may be present on the day of injury.) If symptoms are new and present, there is no lower limit symptom score. Any score > 0 indicates positive symptom history.
4. **Exertion:** Inquire whether any symptoms worsen with physical (e.g., running, climbing stairs, bike riding) and/or cognitive (e.g., academic studies, multi-tasking at work, reading or other tasks requiring focused concentration) exertion. Clinicians should be aware that symptoms will typically worsen or re-emerge with exertion, indicating incomplete recovery. Over-exertion may protract recovery.
5. **Overall Rating:** Determine how different the person is acting from their usual self. Circle "0" (Normal) to "6" (Very Different).

C. Risk Factors for Protracted Recovery: Assess the following risk factors as possible complicating factors in the recovery process.
1. **Concussion history:** Assess the number and date(s) of prior concussions, the duration of symptoms for each injury, and whether less biomechanical force resulted in re-injury. Research indicates that cognitive and symptom effects of concussion may be cumulative, especially if there is minimal duration of time between injuries and less biomechanical force results in subsequent concussion (which may indicate incomplete recovery from initial trauma).[4-8]
2. **Headache history:** Assess personal and/or family history of diagnosis/treatment for headaches. Research indicates headache (migraine in particular) can result in protracted recovery from concussion.[8-11]
3. **Developmental history:** Assess history of learning disabilities, Attention-Deficit/Hyperactivity Disorder or other developmental disorders. Research indicates that there is the possibility of a longer period of recovery with these conditions.[12]
4. **Psychiatric history:** Assess for history of depression/mood disorder, anxiety, and/or sleep disorder.[13-16]

D. Red Flags: The patient should be carefully observed over the first 24-48 hours for these serious signs. Red flags are to be assessed as possible signs of deteriorating neurological functioning. Any positive report should prompt strong consideration of referral for emergency medical evaluation (e.g. CT Scan to rule out intracranial bleed or other structural pathology).[17]

E. Diagnosis: The following ICD diagnostic codes may be applicable.

850.0 (Concussion, with no loss of consciousness) – Positive injury description with evidence of forcible direct/ indirect blow to the head (A1a); plus evidence of active symptoms (B) of any type and number related to the trauma (Total Symptom Score >0); no evidence of LOC (A5), skull fracture or intracranial injury (A1b).

850.1 (Concussion, with brief loss of consciousness < 1 hour) – Positive injury description with evidence of forcible direct/ indirect blow to the head (A1a); plus evidence of active symptoms (B) of any type and number related to the trauma (Total Symptom Score >0); positive evidence of LOC (A5), skull fracture or intracranial injury (A1b).

850.9 (Concussion, unspecified) – Positive injury description with evidence of forcible direct/ indirect blow to the head (A1a); plus evidence of active symptoms (B) of any type and number related to the trauma (Total Symptom Score >0); unclear/unknown injury details; unclear evidence of LOC (A5), no skull fracture or intracranial injury.

Other Diagnoses – If the patient presents with a positive injury description and associated symptoms, but additional evidence of intracranial injury (A 1b) such as from neuroimaging, a moderate TBI and the diagnostic category of 854 (Intracranial injury) should be considered.

F. Follow-Up Action Plan: Develop a follow-up plan of action for symptomatic patients. The physician/clinician may decide to (1) monitor the patient in the office or (2) refer them to a specialist. Serial evaluation of the concussion is critical as symptoms may resolve, worsen, or ebb and flow depending upon many factors (e.g., cognitive/physical exertion, comorbidities). Referral to a specialist can be particularly valuable to help manage certain aspects of the patient's condition. (Physician/Clinician should also complete the ACE Care Plan included in this tool kit.)
1. **Physician/Clinician serial monitoring** – Particularly appropriate if number and severity of symptoms are steadily decreasing over time and/or fully resolve within 3-5 days. If steady reduction is not evident, referral to a specialist is warranted.
2. **Referral to a specialist** – Appropriate if symptom reduction is not evident in 3-5 days, or sooner if symptom profile is concerning in type/severity.
   - Neuropsychological Testing can provide valuable information to help assess a patient's brain function and impairment and assist with treatment planning, such as return to play decisions.
   - Physician Evaluation is particularly relevant for medical evaluation and management of concussion. It is also critical for evaluating and managing focal neurologic, sensory, vestibular, and motor concerns. It may be useful for medication management (e.g., headaches, sleep disturbance, depression) if post-concussive problems persist.

Figure 4.1. Acute Concussion Evaluation (ACE). Unlimited use granted for clinical and educational purposes. Centers for Disease Control and Prevention: Heads Up. Retrieved from www.cdc.gov/HEADSUP

plan. Originally designed for medical providers, this form could be administered by the school psychologist or school nurse. It is more comprehensive than the Concussion Signs and Symptoms Checklist.

NEUROCOGNITIVE COMPUTERIZED TESTING

Preseason baseline testing is used in many school districts with their student athlete population. The most widely used instrument is *Immediate Post-Concussion Assessment and Cognitive Testing* (ImPACT, 2013). This is a 20-minute computerized assessment of neurocognitive abilities. Student athletes take the assessment preseason to document a baseline score. This provides a reference point for how the student athlete's brain functions when it is healthy.

Several additional computerized neurocognitive tests on the market include CogSport (also known as Axon), Concussion Vital Signs, King-Devick Test for Concussions, and ANAM4 (Automated Neuropsychological Assessment Metrics, Version 4). The neurocognitive test monitors are typically athletic trainers, school nurses, athletic directors, team physicians, or psychologists—all professionals who should be designated as members of the school-based concussion team. These tests are relatively inexpensive, unobtrusive, and easy to administer.

The computerized neurocognitive assessment typically measures player symptoms, verbal/visual memory, attention span (sustained and selective), working memory, processing speed, response variability, nonverbal problem solving, and reaction time. If a student sustains a concussion, he or she can take the test again to compare the data to baseline scores. This helps determine the extent of the injury and to what degree recovery of cognitive processes postconcussion has occurred. Without an established baseline, managing a concussion can be difficult and involves more subjective guesswork. For example, if a student who sustained a concussion only takes a neurocognitive test after the concussion, but there is no baseline—the student's "average" score may be taken as an indicator that the concussion has resolved. However, an established baseline may yield scores that were well above average. Thus, for such a student, an average score is a precipitous drop and indicates that the injury is still affecting cognition.

Although neurocognitive tests can be valuable tools, there are a few drawbacks. First, neurocognitive assessment is not recommended during the acute states of recovery because the cognitive stress of taking the test can slow recovery. While the student is symptomatic, the actual process of taking the test can make symptoms worse. Another issue is that student athletes may know what this test is for and sometimes will "fake bad" during baseline so they are not sidelined during future games and practices due to a drop in scores. Next, the most common baseline test, ImPACT, does not test balance or vision, two brain functions that can be key indicators of concussion.

Neurocognitive assessments should only be one of multiple tools used in making return-to-play decisions. Other tools may include an evaluation about conditions that affect concussion recovery, past concussion history, a symptom checklist and/or rating scale, and a complete neuropsychological examination, which generally includes balance testing.

SIDELINE ASSESSMENT

Districts may train staff members to use sideline assessment tools at sporting events to determine whether a student athlete may have sustained a concussion. A sideline assessment can provide a quick, objective way of evaluating whether an athlete should be removed from play. Sideline assessments can measure impairments of eye movements, attention, concentration, speech/language, and other correlates of impaired brain function. A more detailed neuropsychological evaluation, administered at a later time, would then be expected to guide return-to-play decisions.

Physicians, athletic trainers, and coaches are typically the ones responsible for determining whether a student athlete may have sustained a concussion and needs to be pulled from the game (following the mantra, "*When in doubt, sit them out.*"). This often involves a series of questions, with the intention of evaluating whether an athlete is oriented and knows what is going on. Inappropriate responses to simple questions, such as "*What play were you were injured on?*" "*What's the score?*" and "*What do you remember about what just happened?*" help discern whether the athlete is alert to his or her surroundings and circumstances. The athletic and medical team may also conduct simple cognitive tests at the sidelines, such as having the student athlete repeat a series of digits forward and backward and completing simple balance tests. These may look similar to tests a police officer would give to someone suspected of drinking and driving: *Can the person stand with feet in a heel-to-toe tandem position? Can the person stand on one foot? Can the person do that with his or her eyes open and then closed? With his or her hands on hips?* The evaluator must take particular care when conducting informal sideline assessments with very young children, who may not understand slang terminology, such as getting their "bell rung," and who may not even pay attention to the score of the game.

Screening tools such as the Sport Concussion Assessment Tool-3 (SCAT3), Standardized Assessment of Concussion (SAC), or Balance Error Scoring System (BESS) are frequently used sideline assessment tools. Such sideline assessments do have their share of false positives (pulling an athlete out of a game for a concussion when the athlete did not have one) and false negatives (not suspecting a concussion when the athlete actually had one). Symptoms of other conditions, such as dehydration, can mimic the symptoms of concussion. Thus, a brief sideline assessment cannot replace comprehensive testing or be used alone for concussion management. The following are examples of sideline assessments:

Sport Concussion Assessment Tool (SCAT3) and Child SCAT3 (McCrory et al., 2013a, 2013b)

- Compilation of Glasgow Coma Scale (GCS; Teasdale and Jennett, 1974), which measures the degree of brain impairment, the BESS (described in the following), a symptom checklist, and a neck evaluation
- Athlete documentation: Asks the player to report symptom severity on a chart; provides a list of signs to watch for and provides an explanation of what to expect postconcussion
- Medical evaluation documentation: Asks about signs experienced by the player; provides memory questions (e.g., *What team did we play last? Which half is it? Who scored last?*); includes cognitive assessment (five word recall, in which both immediate and delayed responses are tallied); conducts a neurologic screening (speech, eye motion and pupils, gait); provides an explanation of return to play guidelines

Balance Error Scoring System (BESS) (Riemann, Guskiewicz, & Shields, 1999)

- Three 20-second balance tests performed on firm surface and piece of medium-density foam, with eyes closed
- The balance test positions include: standing flat on both feet with hands placed on the iliac crests, standing on a single leg on the nondominant foot, and standing flat on both feet with eyes closed
- Measures central integration of vestibular, visual, and somatosensory information

Standardized Assessment of Concussion (SAC) (McCrea, Kelly, & Randolph, 2000)
- Designed to take 5 to 10 minutes to administer
- Measures orientation, memory, concentration, and delayed recall
- Also includes a brief neurological screen (loss of consciousness, posttraumatic amnesia, coordination, movement)

King-Devick Test (Galetta et al., 2011)
- Two-minute test based on the time to perform rapid number naming
- Requires athletes to read single digit numbers on a tablet. Involves reading aloud a series of single digit numbers from left to right. Scores are compared to baseline
- Screens for saccadic eye movements, attention, concentration, speech/language, and other correlates of suboptimal brain function

SMARTPHONE AND TABLET APPS

A number of concussion apps are increasingly available on the market. They generally offer a quick and easy way to assess youth for a suspected concussion. Many of these apps target parents and coaches, who would both benefit from having the lists of concussion signs and symptoms at their fingertips—on their phone that is always with them—as opposed to on a paper handout in the filing cabinet. While these apps can be quite convenient, it is important that they not be used as substitutes for comprehensive training on the signs and symptoms of concussion, as well as the danger signs. The following list is just a sampling of resources that are available for a smartphone or tablet.

- ***CDC "Heads Up" App, Version 1.0*** (CDC, 2015). Aids in the detection of concussion and provides guidance on what to do if a concussion is suspected. Includes a three-dimensional helmet feature to help parents select and appropriately fit helmets for a variety of sports. The app includes a section on safety tips to prevent injuries at home, school, and play.
- ***PAR's Concussion Recognition and Response: Coach and Parent Version, Version 1.2.2*** (Gioia, Mihalik, & PAR, Inc., 2011). This app, designed by two of the leaders in the field of youth sports concussion, provides a checklist of concussion signs/symptoms designed to help coaches/parents determine whether to remove

a child from the game/practice and seek a medical evaluation. Coaches can immediately e-mail a report of student concussion symptoms generated from the checklist; the app also features a "Dial 911" button for emergency situations and offers strategies for managing concussion beyond the acute phase of injury. The app contains six sections: Past Incidents; New Incident; Home Symptom Monitoring; Concussion Info/FAQs; ACE Post-Concussion Home/School Instructions; and Return-to-Play Guide.

- *Play It Safe Concussion Assessment, Version 1.3* (Concussion Health, LLC, 2011). *Play It Safe* provides a simplified symptom checklist, Maddock's Questions (orientation to time and space), word recall test, number reversal test, balance test, and vision test. The app includes a Dynamic Vision Test, which tests the vestibular ocular reflex. It also includes an established eye chart baseline and measures the subject's ability to read the eye chart while moving their head.
- *ImPACT, Version 1.0* (ImPACT Applications, Inc., 2013). This application is designed to help identify concussion signs and symptoms at the site of a potential injury. It consists of brief cognitive tests and a symptom inventory on which the student is asked to rate severity of concussion symptoms.
- *Return2Play, Version 1.5* (The University of Michigan, 2013). This app is used primarily by patients to track their recovery. It includes concussion myths and facts, signs and symptoms, what to do during recovery, return-to-play guidelines, a list of factors that may increase risk of concussion, and information on how to reduce concussion risk.
- *American Academy of Neurology's Concussion Quick Check, Version 2.2.0* (American Academy of Neurology, 2015). The Quick Check is designed to help parents/coaches and other nonmedical personnel determine if an athlete has a concussion and needs a medical evaluation. It contains a list of common signs and symptoms; a checklist of things to do if the athlete is knocked unconscious (check ABCs); a list of things to do if a concussion is suspected; and a brief discussion on return-to-play guidelines.
- *King-Devick Test, Version 1.0* (King-Devick, LLC, 2015). The King-Devick Test, described under "sideline assessments" presented earlier, can also be administered by parents. The King-Devick Test is a 2-minute test that requires an athlete to read single digit numbers displayed on a tablet or on an iPad. An athlete is given the test at baseline and again after a suspected concussion.

If the time required to complete the test is any longer than the athlete's baseline test time, it is recommended that the athlete be removed from play and evaluated by a licensed professional.

Julia

Julia's coach conducted a sideline assessment at the soccer game in which she sustained her third concussion. After Julia was elbowed in the head by another player, she fell to the ground. Her coach administered the SAC to evaluate her orientation, immediate memory, and neurologic state. Julia was confused about the day of the week and time. She could not recall what happened right before and after the injury. She also appeared uncoordinated and weak. She had difficulty with immediate and delayed word recall, as well as ability to concentrate, as evidence by her impaired ability to repeat strings of digits or state the months of the year in reverse. Because of this assessment, Julia's coach felt confident in her decision to pull her from the rest of the game and to refer her for an evaluation by a medical professional.

CLINICAL EVALUATION

Neurocognitive tests, sideline assessments, and smartphone apps can help district staff and parents determine the severity of a student's symptoms. However, they are not a replacement for a complete medical evaluation to diagnose a concussion. Any student suspected of having a concussion should be seen as soon as possible by a health care provider with knowledge and experience in diagnosing concussions. A student who has sustained a concussion should then be under the continued care of a qualified medical professional throughout recovery. Results from any of the tools previously discussed should be provided to parents and to medical personnel to aid in diagnosis and treatment.

The primary tool for concussion diagnosis in a medical setting is confirmation of a constellation of signs and symptoms after an individual has sustained a blow to the head or body. A physician may conduct balance testing and other neurocognitive assessments. He or she may also conduct neuroimaging, and other physical and neurological exams to rule out more serious injuries. A neuropsychological assessment to assess cognitive functioning, memory, speed, and processing time may also be administered. Research on the effectiveness of neuropsychological tests for identifying and managing concussions, however, is mixed (Institute of Medicine & National Research Council, 2014).

ONGOING ASSESSMENT AT SCHOOL

Keeping an eye on a student who has sustained a concussion and collecting data from multiple sources can help safely and effectively manage a student through the course of recovery. Parents can monitor symptoms at home, medical personnel can monitor symptoms at check-ups, and the school team can implement active symptom progress monitoring at school to facilitate data-based decision making. This allows team members to:

- Assess and monitor the effects of cognitive exertion
- Assess key parts of the day/key classes where symptoms worsen
- Gradually withdraw accommodations that are no longer needed
- Guide the overall return-to-learn and return-to-play decisions

Multiple sources of data help to safely assist a student who has sustained a concussion through the recovery process. The multidisciplinary team described in detailed in Chapter 3 lends itself well to facilitating the collection of data from a variety of sources.

Case Management

The CTL should keep track of all concussion cases brought to his or her attention. A simple spreadsheet, such as the one found in Exhibit 4.3, can be used to collect data on each student's grade level, the person who provided notification, the date of injury, the date of referral, concussion details, and response notes. This type of form can be particularly helpful when tracking the progress of a student who has sustained multiple concussions, as it is easy to search by the student's name for cases that were documented in previous years.

Each student recorded on the tracking log would also have a file containing the signed release of information, physician evaluations and recommendations, copies of ongoing symptom monitoring forms, and the academic adjustment plan.

EXHIBIT 4.3

Sample CTL Case Tracking

STUDENT NAME	GRADE	WHO NOTIFIED CTL	DATE OF INJURY	DATE OF REFERRAL	CONCUSSION DETAILS	RESPONSE NOTES
Ben D.	4	Teacher	Sun. 10/18/15	10/21/15	Sustained during tackle in rec. league football game; first year player; no prior concussions	Went to ED 6 hours after the injury; had danger signs; diagnosed with concussion at ED, told to stay home during acute phase. Stayed home 2 days. Also told to follow up with PCP or conc. specialist. This has not yet occurred. Secured ROI; discharge instructions on file. Admin. Symptom log and dev adj plan.

CTL, concussion team leader; ROI, release of information.

Symptom Progress Monitoring

Much of the return to school progression is dependent upon gradually increasing academic work without exacerbating symptoms. However, it can be difficult for teachers to discern how much cognitive exertion is too much, particularly when some teachers may only see students for short academic periods once a day. The team can facilitate a trial-and-error process that evaluates whether symptoms worsen when the task demands change. Teachers should only change one of the following task variables at a time:

1. Amount of work
2. Length of work
3. Difficulty of work

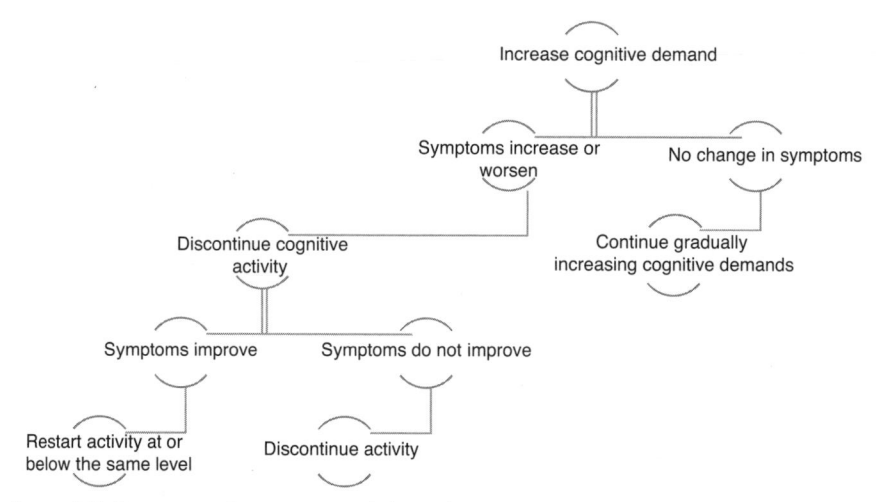

```
                          Increase cognitive demand
                                   |
                    ┌──────────────┴──────────────┐
            Symptoms increase or            No change in symptoms
                  worsen                             |
                    |                      Continue gradually
        Discontinue cognitive              increasing cognitive demands
             activity
                |
        ┌───────┴────────┐
   Symptoms improve   Symptoms do not improve
        |                    |
Restart activity at or   Discontinue activity
below the same level
```

Figure 4.2. Decision tree for increasing task demands.

Adapted from Nationwide Children's Hospital (2012).

Changing only the amount, length, or difficulty of work—one variable at a time—will help the concussion team determine if the increase exacerbates symptoms. As long as symptoms do not worsen, the student can gradually increase engagement in school (see Figure 4.2). However, if symptoms do increase, then the activity should be discontinued for at least 20 minutes and the student should be permitted to rest. If this rest period relieves symptoms, the activity can be attempted again (ideally, below the level that produced symptoms). However, if rest does not relieve symptoms, the student should discontinue activity for the day and reattempt the next day or when symptoms have lessened (Nationwide Children's Hospital, 2012).

Julia

Julia's history teacher, Mrs. Rogers, failed to recognize that taking an entire history exam may be too cognitively taxing for Julia while she was in the acute phase of recovering from her concussion. Mrs. Rogers gave Julia the exam, wished her good luck, and expected her to complete it along with the rest of the class. Consequently, Julia failed the history exam. During the exam, Julia was extremely frustrated because she could not remember the material. She also had trouble focusing—she had a terrible headache and the lights were bothering her. Her poor performance was unusual, as Julia was typically a straight A student. Mrs. Rogers did not adjust the amount, length, or difficulty of the work.

Julia's math teacher, Mrs. Coffman, recognized that Julia should not be required to take an exam in the same environment and in the same amount of time as the other students in her class. Mrs. Coffman arranged for Julia to take the exam in the school counselor's office. Mrs. Coffman also made Julia's exam one third the length of her classmates' test. Julia was able to demonstrate her knowledge and earned an A on the exam because of the adjustments Mrs. Coffman's provided. Decreasing the length of the test allowed Julia to demonstrate her knowledge without undue cognitive exertion.

Progress monitoring tools can allow for careful, individualized clinical assessment and tracking from time of injury. A *Concussion Symptom Tracking Log* (see Exhibit 4.4) is a common way to evaluate the presence and severity of symptoms.

The school team then needs to select classroom adjustments based on the student's specific symptom profile. If a student endorses any symptoms as "severe," it likely warrants a referral to the nurse or parent. Such a student may benefit most from being sent home. Students with mild to moderate symptoms can be permitted to participate in the classroom, with appropriate adjustments. Additional information on the process of selecting and monitoring adjustments is provided in Chapter 6.

Ben

Ben's concussion team completed the symptom tracking log (Exhibit 4.5) beginning with his first day back at school. The tracking log was administered daily upon return to school except on weekends, and then every few days toward the end of this recovery period. His symptoms resolved completely within 3 weeks.

With a quick glance it is clear that Ben's symptoms were primarily cognitive, and that with the exception of a headache, his physical symptoms resolved fairly quickly. He was also tired and sleeping more than usual. His emotional symptoms—which peaked the night after his accident—dissipated by his second day back at school.

Informal Interviews

Interviews can also be used at school to engage a student in dialogue about symptoms. This is particularly helpful because symptoms can vary from day to day, from class to class—and even within a single class session. In-depth conversations with the

EXHIBIT 4.4

Progress Monitoring—Concussion Symptom Tracking Log
Concussion Symptom Tracking Log

Rate on 0-6 intensity scale

0 = not present, 1-2 = mild, 3-4 = moderate, 6 = severe

Symptoms	DATE Day of Injury	DATE	DATE	DATE	DATE	DATE	DATE	DATE	DATE
Cognitive									
Difficulty thinking clearly									
Difficulty concentrating									
Difficulty remembering									
Feeling slowed down									
Feeling sluggish or hazy									
Physical									
Headache									
Nausea									
Vomiting									
Balance problems									
Dizziness									

(continued)

EXHIBIT 4.4

Progress Monitoring—Concussion Symptom Tracking Log (continued)

Symptoms	DATE Day of Injury	DATE	DATE	DATE	DATE	DATE	DATE	DATE	DATE
Fatigue									
Vison changes									
Sensitive to noise									
Sensitive to light									
Numbness or tingling									
Weakness in extremities									
Neck pain									
Emotional									
Irritability									
Sadness									
More emotional than usual									
Nervous									
Sleep									
Sleeping more than usual									
Sleeping less than usual									
Drowsiness									

EXHIBIT 4.5

Ben's Concussion Symptom Tracking Log
Concussion Symptom Tracking Log

Rate on 0-6 intensity scale

0 = not present, 1-2 = mild, 3-4 = moderate, 5 = moderately severe, 6 = severe

Symptoms	DATE Day of Injury 10/18/15	DATE Wednesday 10/21	DATE Thursday 10/22	DATE Friday 10/23	DATE Monday 10/26	DATE Thursday 10/29	DATE Monday 11/2	DATE Thursday 11/5	DATE Wednesday 11/11
Cognitive									
Difficulty thinking clearly	5	4	3	3	3	0	1	0	0
Difficulty concentrating	5	5	4	4	3	2	2	1	0
Difficulty remembering	5	4	4	3	2	2	1	0	0
Feeling slowed down	5	3	2	1	0	0	0	0	0
Feeling sluggish or hazy	5	3	2	1	1	0	0	0	0
Physical									
Headache	6	4	4	3	0	2	0	1	0
Nausea	6	0	0	0	0	0	0	0	0
Vomiting	5	0	0	0	0	0	0	0	0
Balance problems	4	0	0	0	0	0	0	0	0
Dizziness	4	2	1	0	0	0	0	0	0

(continued)

EXHIBIT 4.5

Ben's Concussion Symptom Tracking Log (continued)

Symptoms	DATE Day of Injury 10/18/15	DATE Wednesday 10/21	DATE Thursday 10/22	DATE Friday 10/23	DATE Monday 10/26	DATE Thursday 10/29	DATE Monday 11/2	DATE Thursday 11/5	DATE Wednesday 11/11
Fatigue	5	4	4	3	3	3	1	0	0
Vison changes	0	0	0	0	0	0	0	0	0
Sensitive to noise	4	2	1	0	0	0	0	0	0
Sensitive to light	4	2	1	0	0	0	0	0	0
Numbness or tingling	0	0	0	0	0	0	0	0	0
Weakness in extremities	0	0	0	0	0	0	0	0	0
Neck pain	2	0	0	0	0	0	0	0	0
Emotional									
Irritability	4	2	0	0	0	0	0	0	0
Sadness	4	2	0	0	0	0	0	0	0
More emotional than usual	5	2	0	0	0	0	0	0	0
Nervous	0	0	0	0	0	0	0	0	0
Sleep									
Sleeping more than usual	6	4	4	3	2	1	0	0	0
Sleeping less than usual	0	0	0	0	0	0	0	0	0
Drowsiness	6	4	4	3	2	1	0	0	0

student can help educators target specific barriers to the student's functioning in an academic environment. Open-ended questions might include:

- *How is your headache* (or other specific, bothersome symptom) *today?*
  - Could add a scaling question: *On a scale from 0 to 6 with 0 being "not at all" and 6 being "the worst pain imaginable," how bad is the headache?*
- *Is anything making your headache worse?*
  - Could specify *are ___ (e.g., loud noises or bright lights) making it worse?*
- *Are you having trouble paying attention in class?*
- *Are you having trouble learning new things? Remembering old information?*
  - Can probe to determine whether there are specific content areas in which learning or retrieval of information is most difficult
- *What is most difficult for you at school right now?*
- *How are things going in _____ (insert specific class)?*
  - This can help discern whether the student would benefit from different adjustments in different classes. Perhaps the student has no symptoms or difficulty in math or science but is struggling in Spanish and language arts. In such a case, adjustments might be minimized or removed in certain classes but retained in others.

Questions can be altered based on the student's age and concussion symptoms. For example, instead of asking a very young child, *"Do you have a headache?"* one might ask, *"Does it feel like something is wrapped tightly around your head?"* or instead of *"Do you feel queasy?"* one might ask, *"Do you feel like you might throw up?"* or *"Does your tummy hurt?"*

In considering developmental issues as it relates to our case studies, Julia and Damien could be asked, *"On a scale from 0-6 with 0 being 'no pain' and 6 being 'worst pain imaginable,' how bad is your headache?"* Because they are in Eleventh and eighth grade, Julia and Damien should be able to understand that scale. However, that question may be too difficult for a first- or fourth-grade student to understand. Carly and

Ben could be asked, *"Right now, how bad does your head hurt? Would you say, it doesn't hurt, it kind of hurts, it really hurts, or it really, really hurts?"*

Once the team has determined the areas that are causing the most significant difficulty for students, changes can be made to the plan. Continuous communication with students through these informal interviews can help them continue coursework without over-taxing their healing brain.

Observations

A student may not self-report symptoms if he or she has competing interests. Perhaps the student is anxious to return to sports practice, driving, technology use, or social engagement. Julia may want to get back to schoolwork so she doesn't fall behind, or Damien may simply not want adults worrying about him (or pestering him with questions!). Thus, observations are essential for discerning whether a student's symptoms are worsening. Educators should be on the lookout for the following signs that a concussion may be continuing to affect a student's functioning in school (Nationwide Children's, 2012, p. 10):

- Greater irritability
- Increased problems paying attention or concentrating
- More emotional than normal/emotional reactions that are disproportionate to the situation
- Less ability to cope with emotions than normally
- Increased difficulty learning or remembering new information
- Difficulty organizing tasks
- Increased forgetfulness
- Inappropriate or impulsive behaviors during class
- Repeating himself or herself

Observations can help identify whether there are specific factors that may worsen a student's symptoms. A few key questions included on the CDC's fact sheet, *Returning to School After a Concussion: A Fact Sheet for School Professionals* (CDC, n.d., p. 9), include:

- Do some classes, subjects or tasks appear to pose greater difficulty than others (compared to preconcussion performance)?

- For each class, is there a specific time frame after which the student begins to appear unfocused or fatigued (e.g., headaches worsen after 20 minutes)?
- Is the student's ability to concentrate, read, or work at a normal speed related to the time of day (e.g., the student has increasing difficulty concentrating as the day progresses)?
- Are there specific things in the school or classroom environment that seem to distract the student?
- Are any behavioral problems linked to a specific event, setting, (e.g., bright lights in the cafeteria or loud noises in the hallway), task, or other activity?

Discussion Points

The team can discuss the data, taken together, and determine whether there are factors that exacerbate a student's symptoms and whether steps can be taken to improve those factors. Such issues may include whether there are certain classes or tasks that pose more difficulty than others, whether there is a specific time of day that is most problematic, and whether there are aspects of the school environment that are particularly distracting or difficult (triggers of problems).

Damien

Damien would have benefited from having a school-based concussion team in place prior to his injury to create a more proactive plan. As it stood, the teachers, administrators, and related service personnel learned a great deal about concussions after the fact. The school psychologist was only assigned to the building one day per week and mostly worked on special education evaluations. The school counselor primarily dealt with class scheduling issues and college applications. Both of these school-based mental health providers wanted to offer services, but because of their large caseloads felt confined to traditional roles.

The district had an intern school psychologist who was interested in working with high school age students. The intern had received specific training related to concussion recognition and response during her graduate training and she had a number of resources for parents and teachers. She assisted with Damien's school-based evaluation by observing him in the classroom setting. She also conducted interviews with Damien, his parents, and his teachers to gain a better comparison of his current functioning compared to baseline. Results of these informal assessments indicated that Damien was functioning well below baseline academically. Math and writing were now particularly difficult for Damien. Problems in these subject areas seemed compounded by the fact that both math and language arts were scheduled at the end of the day, when Damien was more fatigued. The cafeteria, hallway, and bus made Damien particularly edgy. These data helped the team create a plan that included switching his math and science classes so he had math in the morning, allowing him to eat lunch in an empty classroom with a friend, and riding to school with his mom or dad instead of on the bus.

The intern school psychologist also wanted Damien to switch classes before or after the rush of students in the hallway—which he had done until his cast was removed—but Damien refused to accept this accommodation that would make him stand out so much from his peers. Instead, he agreed to at least go directly to his next class and take his seat instead of lingering in the hallway until the bell rang.

While school concussion teams generally want to use permanent staff members as core team members, it is also advisable that districts use resources wisely. We may want every district to have school psychologists and school counselors working within the recommended student-to-provider ratios, but this is not happening in many districts. This means that such professionals do not have as many opportunities to engage in prevention and intervention activities. By allowing an intern to take the initiative and assume some of the leadership in this case, under the guidance of her supervisor, this school team engaged in creative problem solving and efficient use of resources. It also provided a good experience for the intern, who gained more confidence in taking on the leadership role. Because of this experience, she made sure her future employees had appropriate concussion management policies and school-based concussion teams in place.

NEWER ASSESSMENT TECHNIQUES: THE FUTURE OF CONCUSSION ASSESSMENT?

Readers are advised to keep abreast of research related to the efficacy of newer imaging techniques at detecting concussions. While typical CT scans and MRIs are generally unremarkable in individuals who have sustained concussions, newer techniques such as magnetic resonance spectroscopy, positron emission tomography, single-photon emission computed tomography, functional magnetic resonance imaging, and diffusion tensor imaging may be used in the future.

The use of serum biomarkers is another area yet to be explored in youth concussions. Following a brain injury, proteins may leak from damaged cells into the cerebrospinal fluid and then cross the blood–brain barrier, entering the bloodstream. While the technology is not yet available to detect and diagnose concussions through newer imaging techniques or serum biomarkers, scientific breakthroughs that allow detection through a medical test may be available in the near future.

REFERENCES

American Academy of Neurology. (2015). Concussion quick check (2.2). [Mobile application software]. Retrieved from https://itunes.apple.com/us/app/concussion-quick-check/id613178630?mt=8

Centers for Disease Control and Prevention. (n.d.). *Returning to school after a concussion: A fact sheet for school professionals.* Retrieved from: http://www.cdc.gov/concussion/pdf/TBI_Returning_to_School-a.pdf

Centers for Disease Control and Prevention. (2015). CDC heads up concussion and helmet safety (1.0). [Mobile application software]. Retrieved from https://itunes.apple.com/us/app/cdc-heads-up-concussion-helmet/id999504040?mt=8

Concussion Health, LLC. (2011). Play it safe concussion assessment (1.3) [Mobile application software]. Retrieved from https://itunes.apple.com/us/app/play-it-safe-concussion-assessment/id441786934?mt=8

Galetta, K. M., Brandes, L. E., Maki, K., Dziemianowicz, M. S., Laudano, E., Allen, M., ... Balcer, L. J. (2011). The King-Devick test and sports-related concussion: Study of a rapid visual screening tool in a collegiate cohort. *Journal of the Neurological Sciences, 309*(1–2), 34–39.

Gioia, G. A., & Collins, M. (2006). *Acute concussion evaluation (ACE): Physician/clinician office version.* Retrieved from http://www.cdc.gov/concussion/headsup/pdf/ace-a.pdf

Gioia, G. A., Mihalik, J., & PAR, Inc. (2011) Concussion assessment & response: Coach and parent version (1.1). [Mobile application software]. Retrieved from https://itunes.apple.com/us/app/concussion-assessment-response/id495161270?mt=8

ImPACT Applications, Inc. (2013). Sideline impact (1.0). [Mobile application software]. Retrieved from https://itunes.apple.com/us/app/sideline-impact/id660066713?mt=8

ImPACT (Immediate Post-Concussion Assessment and Cognitive Testing). (2013). The ImPACT test. http://www.impacttest.com/about/. Accessed September 20, 2015.

Institute of Medicine (IOM) and National Research Council (2014). *Sports-related concussions in youth: Improving the science, changing the culture.* Washington, DC: The National Academies Press.

King-Devick Test, LLC. (2015). King-Devick test in association with mayo clinic (1.0). [Mobile application software]. Retrieved from https://itunes.apple.com/us/app/king-devick-test-in-association/id1033607954?mt=8

McCrea, M., Kelly, J. P., & Randolph, C. (2000). *Standardized assessment of concussion (SAC): Manual for administration, scoring, and interpretation* (2nd ed.). Waukesha, WI: CNS Inc.

McCrory, P., Meeuwisse, W. H., Aubry, M., Cantu, B., Dvorak, J., Echemendia, R. J., ... Turner, M. (2013a). Child-SCAT3. *British Journal of Sports Medicine, 47*(5), 263–266.

McCrory, P., Meeuwisse, W. H., Aubry, M., Cantu, B., Dvorak, J., Echemendia, R. J., ... Turner, M. (2013b). SCAT3. *British Journal of Sports Medicine, 47*(5), 259–262.

Nationwide Children's Hospital. (2012). *An educator's guide to concussions in the classroom* (2nd ed.) Retrieved from http://www.nationwidechildrens.org/concussions-in-the-classroom

Riemann, B. L., Guskiewicz, K. M., & Shields, E. W. (1999). Relationship between clinical and forceplate measures of postural stability. *Journal of Sport Rehabilitation, 8*(2), 71–82.

Teasdale, G., & Jennett, B. (1974). Assessment of coma and impaired consciousness: A practical scale. *Lancet, 304*(7872), 81–84. doi: dx.doi.org/10.1016/S0140-6736(74)91639-0.

The University of Michigan. (2013). Return2Play for concussion (1.5). [Mobile application software]. Retrieved from https://itunes.apple.com/us/app/return2play-for-concussion/id555361650?mt=8

# CHAPTER 5

Recovery: Return to Academics, Return to Play

This chapter focuses on the recovery process, emphasizing the importance of both physical and cognitive rest. This chapter also highlights the importance of communication and collaboration—and having a clear plan—before the student with a concussion returns to school. The chapter opens with a section on recovery in the first days following a concussion, including removal from play for athletes and an overall limitation of activities for all students with concussions. The next part of the chapter describes recovery in the first weeks, including the importance of both cognitive and physical rest. Other treatments are described as well.

Next, return-to-school and return-to-play progressions are described, along with a discussion of how to determine when students are ready to return to academic and physical activities. These will be differentiated, as students can return to school while they still exhibit symptoms as long as symptoms are mild and are not exacerbated by school demands, and as long as the school creates a community of caring around that student. However, athletes should not return to play until they are asymptomatic and cleared by a medical professional. This is because, during the recovery period, students who have sustained concussions are extremely vulnerable and at high risk for further brain injury (Shrey, Griesback, & Giza, 2011).

Most students who sustain concussions will recover without complication. Some take less than a week to recover, most take 1 to 3 weeks to recover, and some can take months or years. An estimated 80% to 90% of concussions resolve in 1 to 3 weeks without long-term effects (Collins, Lovell, Iverson, Ide, & Maroon, 2006). Because the rate of recovery can vary a great deal from student to student, plans for returning students to the classroom and extracurricular activities must be individualized. Some students may progress through the return-to-academics stages rather quickly, easily tolerating cognitive activity, whereas others may only be able to tolerate a few minutes of cognitive activity in the days following injury. Because of this, it is essential that the school team conduct ongoing symptom monitoring and include input from the student.

RECOVERY: FIRST DAYS

The disrupted brain cells quickly and naturally begin to reregulate after a concussion. A physician will often recommend very limited activity during this initial phase of concussion recovery. The first 48 to 72 hours are a critical time period for monitoring physical symptoms. If symptoms such as headache, confusion, disorientation, or vomiting worsen, or if the child has significant difficulty waking, it may be a sign of a more serious medical condition developing in the brain and medical attention should be sought immediately.

Removal from play

If a coach or other school personnel suspect a child has sustained a concussion following an observed, reported, or suspected blow to the head or body in a game, practice, or other activity—including in the classroom—the adult should immediately remove the student from the activity and prevent the child from initiating other physical activity. It is important to keep in mind that "play" is not limited to athletic activity. Play includes physical education class, active play at recess, dancing, and so forth. This is the case even if the injury did not happen at school. If a student, parent, or medical provider reports a fall or accident that resulted in a concussion, the school should follow the same "removal from play" procedure and convene the concussion management team. Sideline assessments that can aid in removal from play decisions were described in Chapter 4.

Limited activities

Within days, most children and adolescents who have been diagnosed with a concussion will be ready to attempt an increasing number of daily living activities. As symptoms decrease in number and become less intense, the student can return to school with appropriate adjustments to the school environment (Halstead et al., 2013).

In the first days following a concussion, the student will likely be advised by his or her physician to rest the brain and get plenty of good sleep. He or she should avoid over-exertion to the brain or body. There should be no additional forces: physical, emotional, or cognitive. The student should avoid any activities that produce or exacerbate symptoms, particularly the use of technology and anything that is visually stimulating or at a loud volume. Exertion and rest can be seen as falling along a continuum of activity from no activity/full rest to full activity/no rest. In the first days of concussion recovery, the student's activity should be much more toward the "no activity/full rest" end of the continuum.

RECOVERY: FIRST WEEKS

In the first 1 to 3 weeks following a concussion, the channels in the brain cells continue to reregulate themselves. This process is likely improved if the individual is getting adequate rest and is avoiding activities that flare or exacerbate symptoms. Thus, reporting and monitoring of these symptoms are crucial for evaluating how well the concussion is resolving.

The student should be getting adequate sleep at night. Parents should monitor their child to make sure there are no late nights or overnights. It is helpful if the child can maintain the same bedtime both on weekdays and weekends. Naps and rest breaks during the day can be helpful if the child becomes tired or fatigued, unless they interfere with the child's bedtime. Adequate food and hydration are also important. This includes eating a healthy diet and drinking plenty of water.

In this early phase of recovery, the child should limit both physical and cognitive activity, as these typically cause symptoms to flare and recovery to be prolonged. Physical activity includes sports practice or games, physical education class, physical activity at recess, exercising, and lifting heavy objects or armloads of things. Cognitive activity includes both schoolwork and job-related mental activity, including reading, writing, math, new learning, and heavy concentration. As symptoms dissipate, both cognitive and physical activities can be gradually increased, with careful monitoring for return of signs or symptoms. If symptoms worsen, the student should scale back on both physical and cognitive activities.

Emotional signs and symptoms may be prominent during the first weeks of recovery, as the student may feel "off" and edgy. The student may also be frustrated by missing sports practice, school assignments, and social events. Older students should not be driving while their symptoms are significant, which can lead to additional frustration. School staff should monitor for signs of depression and anxiety.

Cognitive rest

Cognitive rest is considered to be a crucial aspect of concussion management, yet it is often the most neglected (McCrory et al., 2009). Cognitive rest requires avoiding activities that might trigger symptoms. This includes schoolwork and technology, such as television, videogames, and computers. While *full* cognitive rest is really not practical or likely, except when sleeping, the goal is to *limit* cognitive activity to a level that is tolerable and does not exacerbate or cause the reemergence of symptoms. The student should then gradually return to these activities as symptoms dissipate (Arbogast et al., 2013).

This break from activities can be challenging for students of all ages because it requires avoidance of activities that typically comprise a significant part of their daily routines and interactions (Sady, Vaughan, & Gioia, 2011). Staying home from school during recovery is not always helpful because most students who stay home spend a great deal of time using a computer, texting, playing video games, watching television, and listening to music via headphones. All of these activities make the brain work harder to process information and can exacerbate symptoms, thereby slowing recovery. Thus, if a student stays home, he or she must limit such activities. Students who are accustomed to being on the go or continually connected to social media may find it difficult to reduce their involvement in extracurricular activities and constant communication with peers. However, such a break can be immensely beneficial during concussion recovery because brain cells are much more vulnerable to further injury once an initial injury has occurred (Cantu, 2001).

A recent study indicated that increased cognitive activity was associated with prolonged recovery from concussion (Brown et al., 2014). Participants in the study were adolescents who sustained sport-related concussions. Those who continued to engage in full cognitive activity after sustaining a concussion took from two to five times longer to recover on average than those who limited cognitive exertion, as measured by duration of concussion-related symptoms. Those who engaged in the most cognitive activity took approximately 100 days on average to recover, compared to 20 to 50 days for those who limited cognitive activity.

In the aftermath of so much media attention on concussions, however, some treatment teams have swayed too far in the "no activity" direction and essentially advocate for concussed students to shut themselves in a dark, quiet room until they are fully recovered. This likely keeps the students from getting better as quickly as they might if they were engaging in measured doses of cognitive and physical activity (Thomas, Apps, Hoffmann, McCrea, & Hammeke, 2015). Essentially, cognitive rest includes reducing thinking and reasoning to the extent that it does not provoke symptoms. Guidelines for physical rest are similar.

Physical rest

A primary recommendation during the early weeks of recovery is physical rest. The child should have no participation in any physical activity until cleared by a physician, including physical education and sport activities. This is because physical activity after a concussion often magnifies already existing symptoms. There is also the risk of second impact syndrome, as discussed in Chapter 2.

Julia

In the first week after her third concussion, Julia's symptoms were severe. Any physical activity beyond walking around her house triggered a headache. She could not concentrate on reading for more than a couple of minutes at a time. She longed to watch movies on her computer, to listen to her favorite music, and to interact on social media with her friends.

One night Julia's mom went to check on her and found her under the covers listening to music through headphones and checking social media on her smartphone. She talked with Julia about how the bright light in the dark room, plus the interference with sleep, could trigger her symptoms and prolong her recovery. They also discussed how listening to loud music—especially through headphones—tended to exacerbate Julia's headaches. Her parents had already put Julia's computer away and now decided to keep her phone in the kitchen, where she could use it occasionally while being monitored. They also decided to hook up Julia's iPod to speakers in the kitchen so she could still listen to her music, but at a lower volume and with monitoring from her parents.

Other treatments

While Chapter 6 gives extensive coverage to school-based adjustments and modifications that can aid students through the recovery process, adjunctive therapies may be provided to students with concussions outside of the school setting. More research is needed on the efficacy of such treatments, but it is important that school professionals become familiar with them.

Prescription medications

Prescription drugs are sometimes used for patients who are not responding to cognitive and physical rest alone. However, medication should be used as a last resort, as it will not speed recovery and often has adverse side effects. For example, if a student has sleep disturbances after a concussion, medications that help him or her sleep may exacerbate problems with concentration and daytime alertness. Occasionally, neurostimulants in the methylphenidate group are prescribed to help with concentration or memory issues, but these can also lead to sleep disturbances. Medications commonly used for migraines or tension headaches, including some antidepressants, may be prescribed for headaches. Individuals with persistent depression and anxiety may also be prescribed antidepressants or antianxiety medications.

While school-based professionals are not responsible for making medication recommendations, they may be asked to help monitor effectiveness and side effects, as dosages are often determined by trial and error. Typically a physician will start at the lowest dose that produces no side effects, yet achieves the desired effect.

Over-the-counter medications

Medications that can be purchased without a prescription can be useful as well. For example, melatonin, which is a naturally occurring substance made by the brain, may help patients resume normal sleep patterns (Cantu & Hyman, 2012). Some doctors may advocate for the use of over-the-counter pain relievers; however, these should only be taken with a physician's guidance, as overuse of pain relievers can contribute to postconcussion headaches.

Some have touted the possible benefits of omega-3 fatty acids/DHA supplements (fish oil) for concussion management. However, according to the U.S. Food and Drug Administration, there is currently no scientific evidence to support the use of any dietary supplement to prevent concussions or to reduce postconcussion symptoms.

Nonmedication treatments

Robert Cantu, MD, described several nonmedication treatments that have been useful for athletes seen in his concussion clinic. *Vestibular therapy* involves head and eye exercises if dizziness or balance difficulties are primary symptoms. *Cognitive therapy* can be helpful for thought problems. It provides a set of strategies that are used to challenge negative thoughts. It can also help an individual develop compensatory cognitive strategies, such as memory aids, and it can help individuals develop a better understanding of where breakdowns occur in their cognitive processes. Other types of *counseling* can also be helpful to manage the social–emotional and adjustment issues associated with concussion. *Upper cervical spine physical therapy* can be helpful for pain in the upper neck and the back of the head. *Yoga* can help decrease stress levels and alleviate anxiety. Meditation, biofeedback, and other natural approaches can also aid in stress reduction after a concussion (Cantu & Hyman, 2012).

RETURN-TO-SCHOOL GUIDELINES

A recent study found that about half of individuals who sustained concussions received information regarding return to play but only seldom did they receive information regarding return to school (Arbogast et al., 2013). Thus, there may be a widespread lack of understanding related to how a concussion can affect one's academic performance. There are currently not established procedures regarding return to school because it is an individualized process.

Generally speaking, students who have sustained concussions and are in the recovery process can participate in academic activities, but only if appropriate adjustments or accommodations are in place (McAvoy, 2012). A child's "job" is learning and acquiring knowledge, both academically and socially, and school provides the opportunity to practice emerging skills. The process of cognitive exertion is essential to new learning, but we now know that this can possibly exacerbate concussion symptoms and prolong recovery. Thus, school personnel need guidelines on how to best return students to the school environment and how to give measured doses of cognitive exertion that do not cause symptoms to flare. Unfortunately, the academic challenges many students face postconcussion are beyond the school staff's training and knowledge. This results in students who struggle with focusing on academic assignments, who have new mood swings and emotional reactions, who have trouble with memory or new learning, and who are not fully engaged in class activities. Furthermore, without teachers pulling back the reins and enforcing a step-wise return to learn process, students often decide to persevere in their studies despite their symptoms. This is typically because they believe the stress of make-up work or missing important classes will be worse than the symptoms themselves (Sady, Vaughan, & Gioia, 2011).

It is important for educators to monitor a concussed student's post-injury workload and to set boundaries if the student is unwilling to take breaks to rest his or her brain. Parents, medical personnel, and educators can work together with the student to evaluate intensity of symptoms in order to make a decision about returning to school. If symptoms are so severe that the student cannot concentrate on mental activity for even up to 10 minutes at a time, he or she will likely benefit most from staying home on bed rest, with little or no stimulation, including television, videogames, texting, reading, homework, or driving (McAvoy, 2012).

However, if symptoms are tolerable and the student can concentrate on cognitive activity for up to 20 minutes, the student may engage in light mental activity, such as watching one television show or reading a chapter of a book. If such activities exacerbate symptoms, they should be discontinued. As light mental activity is increasingly tolerated, the student can begin to return to school at a level the concussion team agrees upon.

School personnel must also be aware that just because a student may appear symptom free does not necessarily mean that he or she is fully recovered. Therefore, the process of returning to a learning environment, similar to the return-to-play progression, should be gradual. School personnel should watch for (Gioia & Collins, 2006):

- Increased problems paying attention or concentrating
- Longer time needed to complete tasks or assignments
- Increase in symptoms (e.g., headache, fatigue)
- Increased problems remembering or learning new information
- Greater irritability, less tolerance for stressors
- Difficulty managing and completing complex assignments

The student's progressive return to school and full academic participation can be framed in five phases (Nationwide Children's Hospital, 2012b):

Phase 1: No school

In this phase, the student remains at home, first getting full cognitive and physical rest and then progressing to light mental activity as tolerated. In Phase 1, there may be a number of symptoms that prevent the student from being able to participate in school. Physical symptoms may be prominent and interfere with very basic tasks. The body and brain should both rest as much as possible. In addition to no school attendance, the student should avoid activities that may make symptoms worse. These include both passive activities (using computers, texting, video games, television, loud music, etc.) and physical activities (sports practice, running, weight lifting, biking, calisthenics, etc.).

Once the acute postinjury stage has passed, the student can begin light mental activities at home, such as short periods of reading, writing, or watching television. If these activities produce or exacerbate symptoms, they should be stopped. However, as they are increasingly tolerated, the student can progress to the next stage of part-time school attendance.

Phase 2: Part-day attendance

Unlike the return to play progression, a student *can* attend school while still symptomatic as long as the school provides appropriate accommodations. Once the student's symptoms have improved to manageable levels, he or she can begin attending school for half or partial school days. At this stage, symptoms may be exacerbated by complex or lengthy mental activities. Thus, the gradual return to school should be balanced with rest. The student should avoid tasks or triggers that create or worsen symptoms.

The team may advise that the student only focus on core subjects, prioritizing which classes should be attended and which material is a learning priority. Specific adjustments to the school environment and academic expectations must be in place, along with a mechanism for the student to report symptoms. Further, there should be an emphasis on learning at school while allowing for rest outside of school through a reduction or elimination of homework. The school should offer maximum adjustments and include opportunities for the student to take breaks while at school. These adjustments should then gradually be reduced.

Phase 3: Full-day attendance with adjustments

Once the student's symptoms have decreased in severity and number, he or she can resume full-time school attendance. Because symptoms may still be exacerbated by physical or cognitive activity, appropriate adjustments must still be in place. At this stage, one should expect that previous symptom triggers might have a lesser effect on symptom levels. Cognitive demands can gradually increase by adding to the amount, variety, and difficulty of work the student is expected to complete. Part of this involves *prioritizing work*, which is discussed in more detail in Chapter 6.

The school team should continue to prioritize assignments and projects, eliminating unnecessary busy work, and limiting the number of tests the student takes to less than one per day. Homework can gradually increase. There must still be a mechanism through which the student can report symptoms, ideally through the concussion team. Communication within the team is vital at this stage so that accommodations can be reduced and eliminated as symptoms resolve.

Phase 4: Full-day attendance with full academics and no adjustments, but no sports

Once the student has no symptoms, or only mild intermittent symptoms, he or she can attend school full-time with no adjustments. At this stage, the student is expected to be able to fully function without adjustments to the school environment. The team can focus on ways to keep the student's stress level manageable and to help plan whether the student will complete missed schoolwork or whether there are assignments that can remain incomplete without penalty. The student should not engage in physical activity until cleared by a health care professional with experience in diagnosing and managing concussions, such as a physician or athletic trainer.

Phase 5: Full school attendance and participation with full extracurricular involvement

When the student is asymptomatic, both when resting and when engaging in physical activity, full extracurricular involvement can resume. Thus, it is recommended that students with concussions next go through the *return-to-play* progression (discussed later in this chapter) under the guidance of a health care professional.

Carly

Once Carly's school nurse completed the Centers for Disease Control and Prevention (CDC)'s Signs and Symptoms Checklist, Carly's mother had her evaluated for a concussion by her pediatrician. The concussion was confirmed based on the description of the injury and the symptoms reported both at school and at the doctor's office. However, her symptoms were mild enough that Carly's doctor indicated she could go back to school as long as the school implemented a few minor adjustments to accommodate her symptoms. Even though Carly's initial symptoms were not managed as well as they could have been, she was no longer in the acute postinjury phase. Carly's doctor said she could resume light activities at home and as long as those activities did not produce symptoms, she could go back to school the following day, for at least part of the day. Carly's mother called Mrs. Lang and they agreed that Carly would attend school the following day in the morning only. That way Carly could avoid the loud, crowded cafeteria, as well as recess, physical education (PE) class, and the assembly that was scheduled for the next afternoon.

Attending school for a half-day did not make Carly's symptoms worse. The team determined that she would attend school all day the following day and would receive maximum adjustments, including no PE class or active play at recess, no tests, ample rest periods throughout the day, modified assignments, and no technology (including the use of a computer or smartboard). Carly was fatigued at the end of that day and had a mild headache that dissipated with about 20 minutes of rest before dinner. Carly slept well that night and attended school for another full day with the same adjustments she received the previous day. Carly reported no symptoms at the end of that day.

That weekend, Carly rested and engaged in quiet activities. She was not permitted to fully participate in a neighbor's slumber party that she had been planning to attend. She did, however, attend the beginning of the party to give her friend a gift and to have pizza and cake with the other guests.

On Monday, Carly attended school and required only minor adjustments, including no PE class, a reduction of math problems, and the postponement of a reading test. The following day, Carly resumed a full day of school with no adjustments. She continued to feel well and experienced no symptoms. That afternoon, she had an appointment with her doctor to evaluate her concussion symptoms and her progress toward recovery. Carly's doctor cleared her to resume full activities.

The calendar in Exhibit 5.1 shows Carly's recovery process, illustrating a relatively uncomplicated recovery process within a 1-week timeframe.

EXHIBIT 5.1

Carly's Return to Activity Progression

SUNDAY	MONDAY	TUESDAY	WEDNESDAY	THURSDAY	FRIDAY	SATURDAY
	Fell from monkey bars; sustained concussion	Stayed home from school; but did not go to doctor	Attended school half-day	Attended school full day, maximum adjustments. Some symptoms present	Attended school full day, maximum adjustments	Light activity during weekend. No overnight with friend
Light activity	Attended school full day, minimal adjustments	Attended school full day, no adjustments. Doctor cleared her to resume full activity				

RETURN-TO-PLAY GUIDELINES

If a student is still going through the return to school process and is receiving any academic adjustments due to the presence of symptoms, they should not be cleared to return to play. Thus, a successfully completed return to school process needs to occur first.

Guidelines for safely returning a student athlete to play have been established to highlight the importance of physical rest following a concussion. Resuming activities too quickly can increase the risk of subtle neuroinflammation. It is important that schools have clearly articulated policies on *who* can clear an athlete to return to play and *at what rate* they should increase their physical activity. These policies must be in line with the applicable state laws and policies, though district guidelines may be stricter than state laws or policies.

By law in every state, a health care professional has to provide clearance for a student athlete to return to play after being diagnosed with a concussion. This should be a professional with expertise in concussion evaluation and management. Students are generally cleared to return to play when they are symptom-free both at rest and with exertion, symptom-free with no medication, and back to baseline on academics. Some policies also require that student athletes be back to baseline on computerized neurocognitive tests. As described in Chapter 4, athletic trainers or other professionals can conduct baseline testing before the season begins to determine athletes' preinjury levels of functioning. These computerized neurocognitive tests measure factors such as processing speed, memory, and learning.

The Third International Conference on Concussion in Sport, held in Zurich in 2008, resulted in a Consensus Statement on Concussion in Sport (McCrory et al., 2009). This consensus recommended that a student athlete proceed through six steps to return to play. The athlete proceeds to the next level if asymptomatic at the current level for at least 24 hours:

1. No activity, complete physical and cognitive rest
2. Light aerobic activity
3. Sport-specific activities and training
4. Noncontact drills
5. Full-contact practice training after medical clearance
6. Game play

5. RECOVERY: RETURN TO ACADEMICS, RETURN TO PLAY

If symptoms are exacerbated during the six-step progression, the athlete's brain is likely being pushed too hard and he or she should return to the previous stage of physical activity for 24 hours and then attempt the next level again.

Thus, athletes should not be expected to return to play for at least a week after sustaining a concussion. Understandably, this can be a difficult timeline for athletes, coaches, and even parents to adhere to. It can be seen as a disruption to workout or training routines. Athletes might be upset by the thought of letting down teammates or missing out on key competitions. Thus, it is crucial that teammates, family members, athletic trainers, and athletic staff all ensure that athletes are following appropriate return-to-play guidelines and are supported when reporting symptoms. It is important that all individuals understand the potential risks associated with a premature return to play.

Ben

Ben's recreational football league coach, Coach Robertson, was unfamiliar with return-to-play guidelines before Ben's concussion. Once he found out what happened to Ben, Coach Robertson completed online training available through the Centers for Disease Control and Prevention "Heads Up to Youth Sports" program.

Ben's parents had him evaluated at a sports concussion clinic 2 days after he sustained his concussion so they could gain more clear guidance on when he should go back to playing football. Ben continued to complain of symptoms for 2 more days and by the third day he felt better. Under the supervision of his parents and Coach Robertson, Ben gradually resumed activity, first engaging in regular recess and PE class at school and general play at home. When that did not exacerbate his symptoms, Ben went back to practice and participated in some of the light exercises. At the following practice, Ben participated in non-contact drills during the full practice time. That made Ben's symptoms recur, so he sat the next practice out and gradually resumed activity at practice until he could do so without his symptoms recurring. Once Ben could complete full contact practice training without symptoms, he was cleared by his doctor for full game play.

Ben's coach should have been required to complete a more comprehensive training before he began his coaching responsibilities. Some assert that having so many training requirements dissuades volunteer coaches from assuming these roles. Making the trainings easy and accessible to complete can help remove this barrier. Further, most youth recreation league coaches are also parents—and any parent whose child plays youth sports would benefit from learning about the signs and symptoms of concussion, as well as safe return-to-play procedures.

FRIENDS, CLASSMATES, AND TEAMMATES

Much of the discussion related to concussion teams and returning students to the learning and athletic environment has focused on families, academic personnel, athletic personnel, and medical professionals. However, this discussion would not be complete without mention of one important group for school-age children and adolescents—their peer group. Friends, classmates, and teammates can be a crucial source of support for students who are recovering from concussions. They can help by visiting their friend at home, being a good listener, and making the occasional phone call to check in. Once the child is back at school, friends can also help with some of the school-based adjustments, such as eating lunch with the recovering student in a location separate from the cafeteria, carrying loads of books, or doing quiet activities together at recess.

Parents and educators can help by providing accurate and appropriate information to peers about what happened to the injured student and specific ways they can help. It's important for youth to know that even though their friend may look and seem fine, their friend's injury is on the inside and that he or she may be feeling quite sick for a while.

Teammates need to know how to recognize signs and symptoms of concussion both in themselves and in their teammates. They may witness concussive blows on the athletic field that coaches or parents miss. They may hear complaints of concussion symptoms that are not shared with adults. It is important that the entire school community be educated about how to report concussions to the concussion team leader so that comprehensive wrap-around care and progress monitoring can be provided.

Damien

In the aftermath of his car accident and concussion symptoms, Damien was difficult to be around. He was irritable, anxious, and frustrated. Along with his new academic struggles and physical symptoms, there were stressful situations at home. Damien did not freely discuss his problems with anyone.

The intern school psychologist who had conducted some observations and interviews related to Damien's case had become aware of some of these issues. She served as a supportive resource to Damien at school and he came to talk to her when he was feeling edgy or overwhelmed. The intern also helped connect Damien to supportive peers by starting a lunch group for students who shared a similar interest in anime—including Damien.

The intern consulted with Damien's teachers about setting up a "buddy system." She explained that it will be important for Damien to have a few supportive peers to turn to for help if he becomes frustrated during the school day. Damien's teachers knew which peers would be most helpful and supportive for Damien and agreed to initiate the "buddy system" in their classrooms.

REFERENCES

Arbogast, K. B., McGinley, A. D., Master, C. L., Grady, M. F., Robinson, R. L., & Zonfrillo, M. R. (2013). Cognitive rest and school-based recommendations following pediatric concussion: The need for primary care support tools. *Clinical Pediatrics, 52*(5), 397–402. doi: 10.1177/0009922813478160.

Brown, N. J., Mannix, R. C., O'brien, M. J., Gostine, D., Collins, M. W., & Meehan, W. P. III. (2014). Effect of cognitive activity level on duration of post-concussion symptoms. *Pediatrics, 133*(4), e299–e304. doi: 10.1542/peds.2013-2125.

Cantu, R. C. (2001). Posttraumatic retrograde and anterograde amnesia: Pathophysiology and implications in grading and safe return to play. *Journal of Athletic Training, 36*(3), 244–248.

Cantu, R. C., & Hyman, M. (2012). *Concussion and our kids: America's leading expert on how to protect young athletes and keep sports safe.* New York, NY: Houghton Mifflin Harcourt Publishing Company.

Collins, M. W., Lovell, M. R., Iverson, G. L., Ide, T., & Maroon, J. (2006). Examining concussion rates and return to play in high school football players wearing newer helmet technology: A three year prospective cohort study. *Neurosurgery, 58*(2), 275–286. doi: 10.1227/01.NEU.0000200441.92742.46.

Gioia, G. A. & Collins, M. (2006). *Acute concussion evaluation (ACE) and care plan.* Part of the "Heads Up: Brain Injury in Your Practice" tool kit developed by the Centers for Disease Control and Prevention (CDC).

Halstead, M. E., McAvoy, K., Devord, C., Carl, R., Lee, M., Logan, K., ... Council on School Health. (2013). Returning to learning following a concussion. *Pediatrics, 132*(5), 948–957. doi: 10.1542/Peds.2013-2867.

McAvoy, K. (2012). Return to learning: Going back to school following a concussion. *NASP Communique, 40*(6), 23–25.

McCrory, P., Meeuwisse, W., Johnston, K., Dvorak, J., Aubry, M., Molloy, M., & Cantu, R. (2009). Consensus statement on concussion in sports, 3rd international conference on concussion in sport held in Zurich, November 2008. *Clinical Journal of Sport Medicine, 43*(Suppl. 1), i76–i84. doi:10.1136/bjsm.2009.058248.

Nationwide Children's Hospital. (2012a). *A school administrator's guide to academic concussion management.* Retrieved from http://www.nationwidechildrens.org/concussions-in-the-classroom

Nationwide Children's Hospital. (2012b). *An educator's guide to concussions in the classroom.* Retrieved from http://www.nationwidechildrens.org/concussions-in-the-classroom

Sady, M. D., Vaughan, C. G., & Gioia, G. A. (2011). School and the concussed youth: Recommendations for concussion education and management. *Physical Medicine and Rehabilitation Clinics of North America, 22*(4), 701–719. doi:10.1016/j.pmr.2011.08.008.

Shrey, D. W., Griesback, G. S., & Giza, C. C. (2011). The pathophysiology of concussions in youth. *Physical Medicine & Rehabilitation Clinics in North America, 22*(4), 577–602. doi:10.1016/j.pmr.2011.08.002.

Thomas, D. G., Apps, J. N., Hoffmann, R. G., McCrea, M., & Hammeke, T. (2015). Benefits of strict rest after acute concussion: A randomized controlled trial. *Pediatrics, 135*(2), 213–223. doi: 10.1542/peds.2014-0966.

CHAPTER 6

Adjustments to the School Environment

Teachers may receive physician notes indicating that one of their students has sustained a concussion; the physician may recommend academic accommodations. Some notes may be detailed, listing academic accommodations best suited for a particular student and his or her concussion. However, others may provide few details, thereby requiring educators to determine whether the student requires academic assistance and, if so, in what form.

Appropriate environmental and coursework adjustments can be made in a way that allows students with concussion to continue participating in class while also recovering. Students who have sustained concussions typically require short-term adjustments while they are still symptomatic. This chapter opens with a brief discussion of interventions that students who have sustained concussions may receive outside of the school in a rehabilitation setting and at home. Next, appropriate school-based educational plans are discussed in relation to symptom clusters. Extracurricular involvement of students and special grading considerations during recovery are addressed. The chapter also includes guidance to help school teams determine if a child with persistent postconcussion symptoms requires a 504 plan or further evaluation for an individualized education program (IEP). Finally, the chapter concludes with a note on dealing with students who may malinger or continue to report symptoms when they have actually resolved.

INTERVENTION IN A CLINICAL SETTING AND AT HOME

In addition to school-based services, many students who have sustained concussions are actively engaged in rehabilitation in a clinical setting. They may also be receiving medical and pain management in the form of therapy and/or medications. It is helpful when school personnel are fully informed about such treatments so they can provide documentation to other health care providers about any effects—both positive and negative—that are seen at school. For example, a medication may make a student very sluggish at certain points in the school day. Dosage amounts or time of administration may need to be adjusted.

Parents will likely be given recommendations from their child's physician regarding recommendations for rest and recovery at home. Following are a few common home-based recommendations:

- Plenty of rest during the day and plenty of sleep at night.
- No late nights or overnights with friends while symptoms persist.
- Maintain the same bedtime both on weekdays and weekends.
- Encourage daytime naps or rest breaks when your child becomes fatigued.
- Limit activities that require much thinking or concentration. This includes homework, computer work, texting, driving, movies, television, social gatherings, long period of reading, and video games.
- Avoid loud environments and loud music, particularly through earbuds.
- Limit physical activities, particularly those that might result in another blow to the head.

Figure 6.1 is one example of what a care plan, issued by a physician, might look like.

Because the aforementioned activities are what many children spend most of their time doing, parents should also guide their child toward quiet activities that require little cognitive or physical exertion during the acute phase of concussion recovery. A few examples include playing with pets, baking cookies, and visiting with a few friends. With the guidance of a qualified health care professional, parents should monitor their child's symptoms periodically to guide recovery.

It is relatively common for emergency departments to suggest that students with concussions not return to school until they have been seen by or cleared by a health care provider. Such a suggestion can lead to students being out of school for extended periods of time while waiting to be seen by a doctor. This extended time away from school may not be reasonable or necessary (McAvoy, 2012). Medical professionals may also suggest that students not return to school until they are symptom free. While it is advised that students wait until they are symptom free before returning to sports, they do not need to be symptom free to return to school as long as symptoms are not severe and educators make appropriate school-based adjustments to meet the student's needs.

ACUTE CONCUSSION EVALUATION (ACE)
CARE PLAN
Gerard Gioia, PhD[1] & Micky Collins, PhD[2]
[1] Children's National Medical Center
[2] University of Pittsburgh Medical Center

TODAY'S DATE_____ INJURY DATE_____

You have been diagnosed with a concussion, also known as a traumatic brain injury. To prevent further injury, do not return to any high-risk activities (e.g., sports, physical education, driving, etc.) until cleared by a qualified healthcare professional. To promote recovery, **physical and cognitive activity must be carefully managed.** Pay attention to your symptoms (listed below) and avoid too much of any activity that makes your symptoms worse, as this may lengthen your recovery. As symptoms improve, you can increase the level of daily activity slowly and carefully. Children and teenagers will need the help of parents, teachers, coaches, or athletic trainers to help their recovery and return to activities.

Today the following post-concussive symptoms are present (Circle or check).   ___No reported symptoms

Physical		Cognitive	Emotional	Sleep
Headaches	Sensitivity to light	Feeling mentally foggy	Irritability	Drowsiness
Fatigue	Sensitivity to noise	Problems concentrating	Sadness	Sleeping more than usual
Visual problems	Nausea	Problems remembering	Feeling more emotional	Sleeping less than usual
Dizziness	Vomiting	Feeling more slowed down	Nervousness	Trouble falling asleep
Balance Problems	Numbness/ tingling			

Neurocognitive Testing (if applicable)
Attention/ Working Memory: Appropriate __ Impaired__ Variable __
Learning/Memory: Appropriate __ Impaired__ Variable __
Response Speed: Appropriate __ Impaired__ Variable __

Exertional Effects: Do Symptoms Worsen with Activities?
Physical Activity: Yes___   No___   No Opportunity___
Cognitive Activity: Yes___   No___   No Opportunity___

KEY POINTS   **Returning to Daily Activities**
Sleep: Be sure to get adequate sleep at night; no late nights or overnights; keep the same bedtime on weekdays and weekends. Take daytime naps or rest breaks when you feel tired or fatigued, unless they interfere with falling asleep at night.
Activity Level: Limit physical and cognitive (mental) activity: Symptoms typically worsen or return with too much activity. Making symptoms worse may slow down recovery.
 • Physical activity includes physical education, sports practices, weight-training, running, exercising, heavy lifting, etc.
 • Cognitive activity includes heavy concentration, learning, reading or writing (e.g., schoolwork, job-related mental activity).
Symptoms as your Guide: Pay attention to your symptoms. As they get better, increase your activities gradually with careful monitoring for return or worsening of symptoms. Let the worsening and/or return of symptoms be your guide to slow down.
Food and Drink: Maintain adequate hydration (drink lots of fluids) and an appropriate diet during recovery.
Emotions: During recovery, it is normal to feel frustrated, nervous or sad because you do not feel right and your activity is reduced. Seek professional help if you feel unsafe or have thoughts of self-harm.
Driving: You are advised not to drive if you have significant symptoms or cognitive impairment, as these can interfere with safe driving.

KEY POINTS   **Returning to School**
 • Students with symptoms and/or neuropsychological dysfunction after a concussion often need support to perform school-related activities. As symptoms decrease during recovery, these supports may be gradually removed.
 • Inform the teacher(s), school nurse, school psychologist or counselor, and administrator(s) about your injury and symptoms.
 • School personnel should be instructed to watch for:
* increased problems paying attention or concentrating   * increased problems remembering or learning new information
* longer time needed to complete tasks or assignments   * greater irritability, less tolerance for stressors
* increase in symptoms (e.g., headache, fatigue, etc.)   * difficulty managing and completing complex assignments
Based on the above symptoms, the following supports are recommended: (Check all that apply)
__No return to school   Return on (date)_____
__Return to school with following supports. **Monitor above symptoms, as they may increase** with cognitive exertion (mental effort)
 __Shortened day. Recommend ___ hours per day until (date)_____
 __Shortened classes (i.e., rest breaks during classes). Maximum class length: _____ minutes
 __Rest breaks during school day. ____ rest breaks per day. ___ AM ___PM ____As needed/symptoms worsen. _____ minutes
 __Allowances for extended time to complete coursework/assignments and tests
 __Reduced homework load. Maximum length of nightly homework: _____ minutes. 20-30' study, 10-15' rest break.
 __No testing at this time / Modified classroom/ standardized testing - only as symptoms and preparation allow; allow breaks as needed.
 __Meet with guidance counselor/ academic advisor to establish reasonable timeline for make-up work (as symptoms permit).
 __Request meeting of 504 or School Management Team to discuss this plan and coordinate accommodations.

Children's
National Medical Center

KEY POINTS	Returning to Physical Activities
• **Return to exercise carefully.** Ask your healthcare provider whether you are ready to begin exercise. Some exercise may be helpful, while too much may slow down your recovery. Do not engage in any exercise that causes a significant return or worsening of symptoms. • Be sure that the PE teacher, teacher at school recess, coach, and/or athletic trainer are aware of your injury and symptoms and that you are not asked to do activities that put you at risk for additional injury or cause you to over-exert. ___ No physical exercise at this time. ___ Begin physical exercise as indicated below (stop all activities if symptoms return or significantly worsen):	

Day/ date*	Physical Exertional Activity (NON-CONTACT ONLY)
	1. **Low levels** of physical exertion that may include walking, light stationary biking, light weightlifting (lower weight, higher reps, no bench, no squat).
	2. **Moderate levels** of exercise with body/ head movement as tolerated. Includes moderate jogging/ brief running, moderate-intensity stationary biking, moderate-intensity weightlifting (reduced time and/or weight from typical routine).
	3. **Heavy exertion.** You may return to your typical, full level of exercise. This includes sprinting/running, high-intensity stationary biking, regular weightlifting routine, non-contact sport-specific drills (in 3 planes of movement).

* Pay careful attention to your symptoms/ cognitive skills at each stage of exertion. Move to the next level of exertion only if symptoms remain absent at the current level. If your symptoms return, let your health care provider know, and reduce activities to the previous level..

KEY POINTS	Returning to Sports/ Physical Education

• **You should NEVER return to play if you still have ANY symptoms.** There is no return to activities involving risk of re-injury until you are symptom-free and fully recovered. In many states it is the law that you must be cleared by a licensed healthcare provider to return.
• **Do not play sports in PE or at recess** until you are fully recovered and cleared by your healthcare provider.
• It is normal to feel frustrated, sad and even angry because you cannot return to sports right away. With any injury, a full recovery will reduce the chances of getting hurt again. It is better to miss one or two games than the whole season.
___ Do not return to physical education (PE) class   ___ Return to Physical Education on _____
___ Do not return to sports practices/games at this time   Restrictions_____
___ Complete the Gradual Return to Play Protocol under the supervision of an appropriate health care provider (e.g., athletic trainer).
This is typically a 5 step process, involving stages 1, 2, 3 of increasing exercise (described above) and stages 4 and 5 (described below). Allow 24 hours between each stage and assure that you remain symptom free before progressing. Full clearance for return to play requires a careful evaluation by a licensed healthcare provider with knowledge and training in concussion management. Cognitive functions, balance, and symptoms must return to 'normal' before it is safe to return to play.

Referral: Based on today's evaluation, the following referral plan is made:
___ Return to this office for re-evaluation and monitoring   Date/Time_____
___ Neurology___ Behavioral Medicine___ Psychiatry/ Psychology ___ Other:_____
___ Athletic Trainer/ Physical Therapist – Typical Gradual Return to Play Evaluation and Treatment
___ Atypical Recovery: Physical Rehabilitation: Subsymptom Threshold Physical Activity Program   ___ days per week, ___ weeks
___ Other_____

Physician/
Clinician Signature   Gerard A. Gioia, PhD   Christopher G. Vaughan, Psy.D.
                         Pediatric Neuropsychologist   Pediatric Neuropsychologist
                         Director, SCORE Program   SCORE Program

RED FLAGS: Call your doctor or go to your Emergency Department with sudden onset of any of the following			
Headaches that worsen	Look very drowsy, can't be awakened	Can't recognize people or places	Unusual behavior change
Seizures	Repeated vomiting	Increasing confusion	Significant irritability
Neck pain	Slurred speech	Weakness or numbness in arms or legs	Loss of consciousness

The SCORE Program wishes to thank The Child Health Center Board for making this publication possible and for its continuing support.
© Copyright G. Gioia & M. Collins, 2006. 10.2012

Figure 6.1. Acute Concussion Evaluation (ACE) care plan. Centers for Disease Control and Prevention: HeadsUp. Retrieved from www.cdc.gov/HEADSUP

SCHOOL-BASED POSTCONCUSSION PLANS

The concussed brain requires both *physical and mental rest* to recover from the injury. A student's focus and ability to learn can be affected by a concussion. Decreasing cognitive activity through absence from school or shortened class periods can help decrease symptoms and facilitate healing. Further, physical activities after a concussion can magnify existing symptoms and increase the risk of a student sustaining a second concussion before the first has healed. Thus, school-based postconcussion plans should also include provisions to decrease physical activities.

A postconcussion plan uses a particular student's symptoms to inform educational support. It is helpful to "front-load" academic and environmental adjustments and gradually withdraw them as the student's condition improves (Halstead et al., 2013). It is important to keep in mind that students may be reluctant to accept adjustments and will instead push through symptoms to complete work. This may be partially due to the anxiety that is associated with work piling up (Halstead et al., 2013; Sady, Vaughan, & Gioia, 2011). This is not healthy for the student.

Adjustments, accommodations, and modifications

Literature related to returning to school while recovering from concussion often refers to academic *adjustments, accommodations,* or *modifications* during the recovery process. Sometimes these terms are used interchangeably. However, this book primarily uses the term *adjustments*. This is to emphasize the temporary and flexible nature of these changes, whether they are adjustments to the school environment or adjustments in academic expectations (McAvoy, 2012). The terms *accommodation* and *modification* are commonly used in discussions related to Section 504 plans or IEPs. While these plans can sometimes be instituted for students who have sustained concussions, as is discussed in the next chapter, they are not required for all students who are recovering from concussions. Thus, the words *accommodations* and *modifications* are deliberately used sparingly throughout this text.

Some districts may prefer the use of the term "informal accommodations" instead of "adjustments" (reserving the term "formal accommodations" for those implemented with a Section 504 plan). Each reader is encouraged to determine which terms are preferred in their own regions.

General adjustments for most students

Most students who are recovering from a concussion will benefit to some degree from general alterations to their school day and/or work load. Some of these strategies and considerations are described in the follwoing:

Modified schedule

A modified schedule might involve a shortened day or shortened class periods. For some, the modified schedule might mean that the student only attends core classes instead of electives and/or has rest periods during the day. The student may also start the day late, particularly if his or her school starts very early in the morning. A couple of extra hours of sleep may be particularly healing for the student who is recovering from a concussion.

Modified assignments

Because the concussed brain takes longer to process information and must work harder to do so, it is generally best to allow students to postpone assignments and projects or to complete shortened assignments until they feel better. Grades should be based on this adjusted work. Students who feel well enough to take a test should be permitted to have extended time so their brain has sufficient time to process information.

Prioritize work

As much as possible, avoid having work build up. Students who fall behind in their work can become very stressed and frustrated. This, in turn, can lead to exacerbation of symptoms, particularly emotional symptoms. The concussed student's brain is overwhelmed by the significant chore of re-establishing neurochemical equilibrium. This can make catching up on schoolwork impossible. Thus, the school concussion team must decide what is essential and what is not. Once the team has decided what work has to be done, written due dates for each academic task can help the student to prioritize work.

One of the greatest gifts that can be given to concussed students is excusals from unnecessary work (McAvoy & Eagan Brown, n.d.). This means that the work is not building up and that the student will not be penalized for not completing it. Perhaps the student can be permitted to "audit" a class during the recovery period, which means participation without producing work or being graded. This may be appropriate for elective classes. Because middle and high school students typically take multiple classes, it can be very difficult for them to make up all missed work. Thus, nonessential work should be waived to help lighten the workload. Following are suggested ways for determining how to modify a student's work load (Heinz, 2012):

- Excused assignments—not to be made up
- Accountable assignments—responsible for content, not process
- Responsible assignments—must be completed by student and will be graded

Transportation to and from school

In most cases, a student recovering from a concussion should not be permitted to drive. A school bus can be a loud environment with lots of physical jostling. Ideally, a parent or other responsible adult would drive the student to and from school during recovery. If this is not feasible, modifications should be discussed that could be implemented for the bus ride, including riding at the front of the bus, wearing earplugs, and/or having a "buddy" to ensure the student is not shoved or bothered.

No physical activity

This is generally described as physical activity that can increase heart rate; this recommendation includes no physical education (PE) class, no physical play at recess, and no athletic practices or games.

Alternate periods of mental rest with mental exertion

This can ensure that the student is not engaging in prolonged periods of cognitive exertion, which can exacerbate symptoms. The periods of mental exertion can be gradually increased as tolerated.

Avoid noisy and overstimulating environments

Upon return to school, it is generally advised that students avoid settings such as band class, busy hallways, and the loud, bright cafeteria if such environments make symptoms increase. This environmental consideration is discussed in more detail in the physical symptom section.

Carly

Although Carly's concussion recovery was relatively short in duration, her school implemented appropriate adjustments to the school environment during her recovery. She had ample rest time during the school day; her teacher helped her avoid times and places during the day that were loud, bright, and overstimulating. During PE class Carly rested in the nurse's office. During recess, one of Carly's friends read books out loud to her. Carly's mom drove her to and from school for a few days. Mrs. Lang excused Carly from all homework with no penalty and reduced the number of math problems she was asked to complete during class time. Carly was excused from Friday's written spelling test and told to instead practice spelling the words out loud with her friend during a break.

While the aforementioned adjustments and considerations are generally helpful for most students who are recovering from a concussion, it is also important that the concussion team map accommodations onto specific symptom categories (see Exhibit 6.1).

For students with cognitive symptoms

Minimize distractions

Such students should be allowed to take tests in a quiet room. They can also be given preferential seating in the classroom, typically at the front of the classroom where they can be monitored and have fewer distractions.

Break down or limit assignments

To prevent students from becoming cognitively overwhelmed, give them pieces of assignments that can be completed in small chunks of time (this will vary based on the child's age and preinjury level of functioning). Consider providing a short break before giving the next piece of the task. Reduce repetition to maximize cognitive stamina. For example, perhaps a student could complete five math problems instead of 20 covering the same material.

6. ADJUSTMENTS TO THE SCHOOL ENVIRONMENT

EXHIBIT 6.1

Academic Adjustments for Concussions

Using the student's reported symptoms from the Concussion Symptom Log, select appropriate adjustments from the following list		
Student Name_____ Date:_____ Staff Contact:_____	Start Date	End Date
General		
Adjust class schedule (alternate days, shortened day, abbreviated class, late start to the day).		
Modify assignments as follows:		
Allow student to audit class (i.e., participate without producing or grades).		
No physical educaiton classes or physical play at recess until cleared by a health care professional.		
Remove or limit testing and/or high-stakes projects.		
Alternate periods of mental exertion with periods of mental rest.		
Avoid noisy and overstimulating environments (i.e., band).		
Limited exposure to computers screen time, including smart boards.		
The student will be transported to and from school as follows:_____		
Cognitive/Thinking		
Minimize distractions; provide preferential seating in the classroom.		
Reduce class assignments and homework to critical tasks only. Exempt nonessential work. Base grades on adjusted work.		
Provide extended time to complete assignments/tests. Adjust due dates.		
Once the key learning objective has been presented, reduce repetition to maximize cognitive stamina (i.e., assign fewer problems).		
Allow student to demonstrate understanding orally instead of in writing.		

(continued)

EXHIBIT 6.1

Academic Adjustments for Concussions (*continued*)

	Provide written instructions for work that is deemed essential.		
	Provide class notes by teacher or peer. Allow use of smart phone or tape recorder to tape lectures.		
	Allow use of notes for test taking and/or provide other memory supports.		
	Fatigue/Physical		
	Allow time to visit school nurse, psychologist, or counselor for headaches or other symptoms.		
	Allow strategic rest breaks (e.g., 5-10 minutes every 30-45 minutes) during the day.		
	Allow hall passing time before or after crowds have cleared.		
	Additional limits on physical exertion; avoid carrying heavy loads. Designate a peer to carry bag and books in hallway.		
	Allow student to wear sunglasses or hat indoors. Control for light sensitivity (draw blinds, sit away from window).		
	Allow student to study or work in a quiet space away from visual and noise stimulation.		
	Provide a quiet environment to take tests.		
	Allow student to spend lunch/recess in quiet space for rest and control for noise sensitivity.		
	Limit technology, including texting, computers, TV, loud music, and movies.		
	Emotional		
	Develop plan so student can discreetly leave class as needed for rest.		
	Provide a quiet place to allow for destimulation.		
	Keep student engaged in extracurricular activities. Allow student to attend but not fully participate in sports.		
	Encourage student to explore alternative activities of nonphysical nature.		
	Develop an emotional support plan for the student (e.g., identify adult to talk with if feeling overwhelmed).		

Adapted from: brain101.orcasinc.com and http://www.cdc.gov/concussion/headsup/youth.html.

Provide extended time to complete tests and assignments

As mentioned earlier, teachers can excuse certain assignments, and they can adjust due dates or expectations for others.

Avoid substituting mental activities for physical ones

If a child is being excused from physical activity, such as PE class, avoid automatically using that as a time to "make up" school work. Cognitive exertion can be just as exhausting as physical exertion for a student who is recovering from a concussion. Keep in mind the analogy of the student with a broken arm. (If a student had a broken arm and therefore could not complete a lengthy written test, you would not instead have the student play basketball.)

Give written instructions

Processing auditory information and holding information in one's short-term memory can be difficult for many students, particularly those with concussions. Avoid this by giving concise written instructions, or even having the student write the instructions himself or herself.

Emphasize important information

Dense text on a page can be overwhelming. Use highlighting or color coding to emphasize key passages.

Provide other supports for memory

These might include providing class notes or fact sheets, allowing the student to record class sessions, allowing the student to take open-book or open-note tests, or helping the student develop ways to memorize information (e.g., rehearsal, repetition, mnemonic devices).

Provide assistance in the form of people

A student may benefit from the temporary use of a reader, scribe, note taker, and/or tutor.

Facilitate organization

Educators can help students with concussion use a planner, chart, checklist, or device to keep track of due dates and assignments. They can also check whether a student understands expectations by having the student restate information in his or her own words.

Allow alternative methods for demonstrating knowledge

Allow students to demonstrate their understanding of course material by giving oral rather than written responses.

For students with physical symptoms

Avoidance of sensory overload

If a student has sensitivity to light, he or she should be permitted to avoid bright lights by moving the seat away from windows, dimming the lights in a room, or being allowed to wear sunglasses or a hat. If a student has sensitivity to loud noises, he or she should be excused from classes and events with excessive noise, including band/choir, industrial arts class, pep rallies, assemblies, and dances. It can also be helpful to allow the student to eat lunch in a quiet location rather than the loud, bright cafeteria.

Designate a quiet spot

Allow the student time to rest in the school nurse's office or to visit the school counselor if he or she is experiencing symptoms such as headaches. Strategic rest breaks (e.g., 5–10 minutes every 30 minutes) might be scheduled during the day for prevention of symptoms. Provide a quiet environment for taking tests, as well as a quiet work space for studying and completing schoolwork away from visual or noise stimulation.

Limit technology

Students with physical symptoms should also avoid or limit texting, computers, TV, loud music, and movies (especially 3D movies).

Excuse from activities that require exertion

Until physical symptoms have resolved, the student should not participate in gym, sports practice, or carry heavy loads (such as stacks of books).

For students with emotional, behavioral, or social symptoms

Allow breaks from the environment

Allow the student to leave the room without penalty if a situation becomes frustrating or the student becomes emotional. Concussion recovery can be emotionally taxing and the experience of crying in front of classmates can be traumatic for some students.

Encourage seeking help

The school psychologist, counselor, or social worker can be a tremendous source of emotional support for the student during the school day. Make sure the student meets and becomes familiar with this person *before* there is a highly charged emotional situation. Encourage the student to communicate difficulties to his or her parents or another trusted adult.

Monitor peer relations

A student may feel isolated from peers and social networks. School personnel, particularly school psychologists or counselors, can talk with students about these issues and provide support or encouragement. Keep the student engaged in extracurricular activities as appropriate. For example, a student might be permitted to attend, but not fully participate in, sports practice and games.

Encourage alternative activities

Help the student explore activities of a nonphysical nature that can provide social engagement and peer support.

Avoid singling out the student in front of peers

All teachers and concussion team members should be encouraged to provide these adjustments and supports as privately and unobtrusively as possible.

Ben

> The concussion team at Ben's school completed the Concussion Symptom Tracking Log seen in Chapter 4. The following academic adjustments were selected based on the type and duration of symptoms he was

experiencing. Adjustments were generously applied during the first couple of days when symptoms were still mild to moderate; however, during the second and third week of recovery, they were decreased (see Exhibit 6.2).

EXHIBIT 6.2

Ben's Academic Adjustments for Concussions

	Using the student's reported symptoms from the Concussion Symptom Log, select appropriate adjustments from the following list		
	Student Name____ *Ben Davidson* Date: *10/21/15* Staff Contact:____ *Mrs. Ernst* School Counselor_____	Start Date	End Date
	General		
x	Adjust class schedule (alternate days, shortened day, abbreviated class, late start to the day).	10/21	10/23
x	Modified assignments as follows: *shortened assignments, allow alternate ways to show knowledge; excusals from unnecessary work*	10/21	11/5
	Allow student to audit class (i.e., participate without producing or grades).		
x	No physical education classes or physical play at recess until cleared by a health care professional.	10/21	11/11
x	Remove or limit testing and/or high-stakes projects.	10/21	11/5
x	Alternate periods of mental exertion with periods of mental rest.	10/21	11/5
x	Avoid noisy and overstimulating environments (i.e., band).	10/21	10/23
x	Limited exposure to computer screen time, including smart boards	10/21	11/5
x	The student will be transported to and from school as follows: _____ *mom will drive* _____	10/21	10/23
	Cognitive/Thinking		
x	Minimize distractions; provide preferential seating in the classroom.	10/21	11/5
x	Reduce class assignments and homework to critical tasks only. Exempt nonessential work. Base grades on adjusted work.	10/21	11/5

(continued)

EXHIBIT 6.2

Ben's Academic Adjustments for Concussions (*continued*)

x	Provide extended time to complete assignments/tests. Adjust due dates.	10/21	11/5
x	Once key learning objective has been presented, reduce repetition to maximize cognitive stamina (i.e., assign fewer problems).	10/21	11/5
x	Allow student to demonstrate understanding orally instead of in writing.	10/21	11/5
x	Provide written instructions for work that is deemed essential.	10/21	11/5
	Provide class notes by teacher or peer. Allow use of smart phone or tape recorder to tape lectures.		
x	Allow use of notes for test taking and/or provide other memory supports.	10/21	11/5
	Fatigue/Physical		
x	Allow time to visit school nurse, psychologist, or counselor for headaches or other symptoms.	10/21	11/5
x	Allow strategic rest breaks (e.g., 5-10 minutes every 30-45 minutes) during the day.	10/21	10/23
	Allow hall passing time before or after crowds have cleared.		
x	Additional limits on physical exertion; avoid carrying heavy loads. Designate a peer to carry bag and books in hallway.	10/21	11/5
x	Allow student to wear sunglasses or hat indoors. Control for light sensitivity (draw blinds, sit away from window).	10/21	10/23
x	Allow student to study or work in a quiet space away from visual and noise stimulation.	10/21	10/23
x	Provide a quiet environment to take tests. *No tests.*	10/21	10/23
x	Allow student to spend lunch/recess in quiet space for rest and control for noise sensitivity.	10/21	10/23
x	Limit technology, including texting, computers, TV, loud music, and movies.	10/21	11/05
	Emotional		
	Develop plan so student can discretely leave class as needed for rest.		

(*continued*)

EXHIBIT 6.2

Ben's Academic Adjustments for Concussions (*continued*)

x	Provide quiet place to allow for de-stimulation.	10/21	10/23
	Keep student engaged in extracurricular activities. Allow student to attend but not fully participate in sports.		
	Encourage student to explore alternative activities of nonphysical nature.		
	Develop an emotional support plan for the student (e.g., identify adult to talk with if feeling overwhelmed).		

DECISION MAKING DURING RETURN TO ACADEMICS

Learning new material can be very difficult for a student who is recovering from a concussion. This is because the concussed brain is recalibrating neurons that have gone out of whack. Thus, teachers need to be sensitive to the fact that while students need to be accountable for course objectives, the concussed brain is compromised. It is not efficiently processing new learning. Information presented to students while they are recovering from concussions is difficult to convert into memory and conceptualize overall. Educators can allow participation at school to an extent that does not worsen symptoms. As academic adjustments are no longer needed, the concussion team leader (CTL), in collaboration with other members of the concussion management team (CMT), can withdraw a student's academic adjustments. The end date of each adjustment should be noted on the Academic Adjustments for Concussions form.

Cognitive demands can gradually increase as long as there is no change in symptoms. However, if symptoms increase or worsen, the activity should be discontinued and the student should be permitted complete cognitive rest for 20 minutes. If symptoms improve with this rest, the student can restart the activity at or below the same level that produced symptoms (Nationwide Children's Hospital, 2012).

For example, Ben was working on math problems at his desk and began to get a headache. His teacher had him stop working on the math sheet and sent him down to the nurse's office to lie down for 20 minutes and his headache went away. When he returned, he only had five problems left, so his teacher had him complete the sheet and then resume regular activities with the rest of the class.

If the symptoms do not improve even with 20 minutes of rest, the student should discontinue the activity and resume when symptoms have lessened, such as the next day. So, using the aforementioned example, if Ben rested in the nurse's office for 20 minutes and his headache did not improve, he should have been sent home, been allowed to continue to rest in the nurse's office, or perhaps been permitted to return to the classroom for an activity involving less cognitive exertion, such as listening to an audio book or watching his teacher lead a science experiment.

EXTRACURRICULAR INVOLVEMENT DURING RECOVERY

The concussion team may need to discuss the student's extracurricular involvement during the recovery period. It can certainly be upsetting for teachers to put great effort into accommodating the concussed student's needs in the classroom and then see that same student running up and down the bleachers, socializing at a school football game on Friday night while the loud band plays in the background.

Every student's situation varies depending on the student's age, level of involvement with extracurricular activities, and the nature of concussion symptom severity and duration. A blanket policy banning all social activity and extracurricular involvement for prolonged periods of time can exacerbate feelings of depression, anxiety, isolation, and despair.

It might be most helpful to significantly restrict extracurricular involvement—including something as simple as after school meetings —during the acute recovery phase, allowing the student to put all of his or her energy into getting better and performing as well as possible at school. However, if recovery is protracted for weeks or months, it may be beneficial for the student to have some extracurricular involvement added to the recovery plan to keep him or her socially engaged and upbeat.

In such a case, the concussion team might discuss activities in terms of their likelihood of provoking symptoms. Playing percussion in the band might exacerbate headaches, while participating in after school student council meetings might not be a problem. A field trip to an amusement park would not likely be advised, but one to a nature center would not be as likely to provoke symptoms. In such a situation, it would be ideal if a parent could drive the student in order to avoid the bumpy bus ride and also serve as an extra chaperone—not one relied on for supporting other children—so the student could be taken home early if necessary. If there is a once-in-a-lifetime event such as prom or graduation, the concussion team might discuss how the student can participate safely, perhaps by wearing earplugs, attending for a shortened period of time, and not dancing (McAvoy & Eagan Brown, 2015).

SPECIAL GRADING CONSIDERATIONS

Whether a student is newly injured or has been struggling with concussion symptoms for months, it can be difficult for teachers to determine whether to administer exams and how to assign grades. Again, there are no hard and fast rules, but the following considerations can help guide a school team's decisions on this issue.

Regarding exams, it is important that teachers consider the reasons tests are administered. Generally the purpose is both to evaluate a student's mastery of the class material and to facilitate the assignment of a grade for that quarter. When a student is in the acute stages of recovering from a recent concussion, the process of taking an exam might exacerbate symptoms and prolong recovery. Further, because of fatigue and slow processing, an exam is unlikely to yield an accurate representation of the student's knowledge of the subject matter. Additionally, the student may have missed school immediately after injury and may have missed content coverage, thereby leading to gaps in his or her knowledge. Essentially, it might not be fair to test the student on the material and, in fact, it might make symptoms worse.

In such situations, a teacher might consider exempting the student from the midterm or final examination altogether and base the student's grade on work completed prior to the concussion. If insufficient work was completed before the end of the grading period to justify a grade, the teacher might consider another way to evaluate the student's mastery of the course content. For example, instead of taking a lengthy written test, perhaps the student could complete an oral examination or multiple choice test, both of which are less cognitively taxing.

Some students might not want to have their grade based on work completed prior to the concussion because they were hoping to bring their grades up with final exams. Rather than having such students push through a final exam schedule, it might be beneficial to space out exams, allowing for ample rest between tests, and to limit this to only one or two classes.

For students who are struggling with prolonged symptoms or who may have missed a great deal of class and/or received adjustments for months, teachers may question whether they have mastered the course content sufficiently to pass the class. Assigning a grade for such students can be difficult. In such situations, teachers are advised to talk with one another and seek guidance from an administrator and the concussion team. Planning ahead for the last month of instruction can be helpful, as the teacher can determine the essential knowledge required for the student to exit the class. If the student has not received that instruction, the material must be retaught before it can be assessed and graded. McAvoy and Eagan Brown (2015) offer the following strategies on how to do this:

- **Focus** on essential material in the last month before grading
- **Reduce** semiessential material
- **Remove** nonessential material altogether
- **Forget** about "make-up" work unless it is essential to current knowledge

Once the student has received the essential knowledge for course completion, the teacher can then determine the best way to assess that knowledge. Again, it is important to avoid having work build up, as that can be incredibly stressful for students recovering from concussions. Suggestions can be given to the student to help reinforce skills and knowledge, but a report card full of incompletes and work building up from one semester to the next will be counter-productive for concussion recovery.

Damien

Damien missed weeks of instruction after his car accident. Then, once he returned to school, his concussion interfered with his ability to learn new material and to complete work that was on par with his classmates. He had six teachers and, without the guidance and support of a concussion team, they struggled to determine how to assign his grades for the semester.

His English teacher allowed him to do an oral report on *Of Mice and Men* instead of the written report everyone else completed. The class took a test every Friday on sentence structure/compound sentences; the teacher did not count the grades for the tests administered on the days Damien was absent. When he was present, Damien took the tests, which had four multipart questions and took about 20 minutes to complete—and he did well on them. She graded Damien's in-class work on the days he was present, which involved participating in group discussions and answering written and oral questions in class. She provided study guides that had the answers filled in rather than requiring that he complete them as homework. Damien earned a B+ in the class, which was the same grade he had before his car accident.

Damien's history teacher also made appropriate adjustments during his recovery period. Students completed packets in class, which was part of her regular instruction, and did not exacerbate Damien's symptoms. For the final exam, Damien was given a multiple choice test instead of an essay exam. He earned a B in the class.

Damien's science teacher typically had the class do an activity each day, which involved a project with classmates at Damien's table. They completed analysis questions, discussed how the experiment worked, and related their findings to scientific principles. Because much of his science grade was based on these activities, and Damien's teacher had no way of having him make up these activities, Damien's teacher based his grade for this part of the class on the days he was there. This was helpful, as he did well with these hands-on group projects. However, Damien struggled to remember information on the tests and did not consistently turn in his homework. He earned a C in science.

Spanish was difficult for Damien, as it involved a great deal of drill and practice and new learning. There was a great deal of in-class packet work and the prolonged cognitive exertion made his symptoms flare. Damien was expected to complete all the same work as other students, and received no adjustments. He failed his exam and dropped Spanish after the first quarter.

Damien played trombone in the school band. The pressure of blowing into his trombone plus the cacophony of the band was excruciating. Damien almost always ended up with a headache after band class. The class included "challenges" of people in higher chairs and he fell from second chair to last. He dropped band.

His math teacher said that because Damien was at school, he was responsible for all the same work as everyone else—same classwork, same homework, same tests. Damien failed math that quarter.

SPECIAL PLANS FOR STUDENTS WITH PERSISTENT PROBLEMS

Most students only require temporary, informal academic adjustments after a concussion. If managed appropriately, concussion symptoms should resolve within a few weeks. However, the nature of the concussion, the student's history of concussions, and other pre-existing conditions can all affect recovery. Approximately 10% to 20% of students who have sustained concussions may have symptoms that extended beyond 3 or 4 weeks (Collins, Lovell, Iverson, Ide, & Maroon, 2006).

If a student's concussion symptoms persist, academic accommodations and student support may be provided through multi-tiered systems of support, a more formalized health plan, or through options provided under federal law: Section 504 of the Rehabilitation Act of 1973 or, in very rare cases, an IEP under the Individuals with Disabilities in Education Act (IDEA, 2004). The process of qualification and types of plans may vary from state to state.

Multitiered systems of support

A multitiered system of support (MTSS), sometimes referred to as response-to-intervention (RTI), is a stepwise progression of intervention services that allows school professionals to provide interventions of increasing intensity to students who are identified as needing them most. At each level, school professionals use ongoing assessment to determine whether additional support or instruction is needed.

MTSS is a continuum along which student needs are met. By using problem-solving processes, educators can analyze why a student is struggling and determine which interventions are most appropriate.

In concussion cases, the majority of students will be responsive to general short-term academic adjustments. However, some students will continue to experience symptoms that interfere with their educational performance. In such cases, more targeted interventions or academic accommodations (beyond temporary minor "adjustments") may be required. In very rare concussion cases, a disability may be identified that requires intensive supports such as special education services and long-term modification of the curriculum.

Section 504 plans

Because most concussions resolve within a few weeks, short-term adjustments at school can be arranged without the need for a formal 504 plan (Popoli, Burns, Meehan, & Reisner, 2014). However, if a student requires significant academic adjustments for a prolonged period of time or attendance is significantly compromised, the school might consider formalizing adjustments into a Section 504 plan—essentially making the academic adjustments into an accommodation plan (McAvoy, 2012). Accommodations described in a 504 plan would be similar to those described earlier, such as environmental adaptations and behavioral strategies.

Section 504 is part of the Rehabilitation Act of 1973, which was designed to protect the rights of individuals with disabilities in programs and activities that receive federal funding from the U.S. Department of Education. Section 504 requires that school districts provide a free and appropriate public education (FAPE) to students with disabilities regardless of the nature or severity of the disability. This act helps to ensure that students who have disabilities—including disabilities those that are not severe enough to warrant an IEP—receive services and accommodations to meet their educational needs.

Some parents or school teams erroneously believe that a child with a concussion must immediately receive a 504 plan if the child requires accommodations upon return to school. Many students with concussions will not have symptoms of sufficient severity or duration to qualify for a 504 plan. Thus, a medical diagnosis of concussion does not automatically mean that a child should receive a 504 plan. The medical disability must cause substantial limitation to one or more major life activities, such as learning.

If a 504 plan is deemed appropriate for a given student's situation, it is advised that the school concussion team determine which problematic symptoms require accommodations and tailor appropriate interventions accordingly. In such cases, communication among the family, school team, and medical providers must be coordinated, documented, and ongoing—this is a student who is expected to get better and who should eventually no longer require the plan (more information about Section 504 law is available at www2.ed.gov/about/offices/list/ocr/504faq.html).

Julia

Julia's symptoms persisted for 3 months and did not show signs of abating. In collaboration with Julia's parents, her school team ultimately decided to write a 504 plan for Julia, formalizing the adjustments she had been receiving into accommodations (see Exhibit 6.3). Different districts will have different formats and procedures for these plans. Whereas some students' 504 plans for other disorders might be reviewed and revised on an annual basis, Julia's team reviewed her 504 plan monthly because of the expectation that her symptoms would eventually diminish.

EXHIBIT 6.3

Julia's Academic Accommodations With a 504 Plan

Student's Name <u>Julia Martinez</u> DOB <u>4/02/99</u>

School <u>Kennedy High School</u> Parent's Name <u>Rebecca Martinez and Alfonso Perez</u>

Grade <u>11</u> Date of Plan Initiation <u>3/15/16</u>

Sources of Evaluation Information:

Medical diagnosis of concussion–Children's Hospital Medical Center; see attached medical information

Ongoing monitoring of symptoms and results of academic adjustments–Kennedy HS concussion team; see attached

Specify the qualifying physical or mental impairment: Concussion

Check affected major life activities:

___Seeing	___Hearing	___Walking	___Breathing	___Eating
___Sleeping	_X_Learning	_X_Reading	_X_Thinking	_X_Concentrating
___Digestive Functions	___Bladder Functions	___Bowel Functions	___Performing Manual Tasks	___Other _____

Accommodation Needed
No physical education class or vigorous physical activity
Avoidance of loud and overstimulating environments; excused from assemblies, permitted to eat lunch in classroom
Take tests in a separate setting and provide extended time
No more than one test per day
Allow rest breaks in nurse's office without penalty
Reduce class assignments and homework to critical tasks only; exempt nonessential work; base grades on adjusted work
Allow option of demonstrating understanding of material orally rather than in writing when possible
Give paper copies of notes from smartboard or lectures

Individualized education programs

If a disability adversely affects a student's educational performance, that student may be eligible for an IEP under IDEA (2004). Every school district is responsible for finding and identifying students with disabilities; therefore, if the severity and duration of concussion symptoms warrant a full evaluation, the school team might consider eligibility under the special education category of "traumatic brain injury" (TBI). This is preferable to a less specific eligibility category, such as "other health impairment" (OHI), although the team does need to evaluate all areas of suspected need and consider whether alternative classifications might be more appropriate.

Students who are eligible for IEPs under the TBI category may require significant modifications to the curriculum in order to be successful academically. The IEP may include adjustments to a student's workload, instructional delivery, or instructional environment. As such, students may receive part of their instruction in a separate classroom, taught by a special educator. The vast majority of students who sustain concussions will not require an IEP. However, a student who has sustained multiple concussions and thereby sustained permanent impairment may require this level of support.

By implementing an effective plan upon returning to school (including a return to school concussion management protocol and a mechanism for monitoring symptoms to allow for fine-tuning of adjustments), the school team can more easily determine whether a more formal action such as a Section 504 plan or full evaluation under IDEA is warranted (Zirkel & Eagan Brown, 2015).

STUDENTS WHO MALINGER

The vast majority of students who have experienced a concussion have legitimate symptoms and may try to hide how awful they feel. However, a few may exaggerate or feign illness in order to escape work, continue receiving academic adjustments, to get attention, or to avoid resuming their sport. This is made particularly difficult by the fact that concussion symptoms are subjective. Frankly, it can be difficult to know when a student is lying.

If a student has medical documentation of a concussion, he or she should be helped as much as the school is able to provide assistance.

Communication among the concussion team members—all facets, including parents, the medical team, the academic team, and the athletic team—can help identify students who are malingering or trying to take advantage of the situation. If a concern about the legitimacy of a student's reported symptoms arises, the concussion team can meet to determine what steps should be taken. Direct communication among team members—including the student's parents—and documentation by the CTL can be helpful.

Ben

Even though Ben was only in elementary school, his father had great football aspirations for his son. In fact, Ben was never really interested in the sport and played largely to please his father. Although Ben's concussion symptoms had resolved months earlier, at the start of the new practice season, Ben told his mother that his headaches and dizziness had returned.

Ben's mother shared this with the school counselor, Ms. Ernst, who was also the CTL, and asked her to check in with Ben to see if he had additional symptoms that emerged in the classroom. As Ms. Ernst talked with Ben, she realized she was uncovering a problem between Ben and his dad. Ben did not want to play football again. He did not enjoy the sport and he was afraid of being injured again. Through his experiences the previous year, Ben learned that symptoms were a way out of football. When he had headaches and dizziness, he did not have to go to practices or play in games. Ms. Ernst talked more with Ben about how he was feeling and helped him feel safe in his discussion with her.

At one point, Ms. Ernst asked, "Do you enjoy playing football?"

Ben looked down, "Not really."

"Whose idea was it to play last year?" Ms. Ernst asked.

"My dad's," Ben said. "A paper came home from school about it and he saw it on the counter. I wouldn't have asked to do it, but he was real excited. He talked all about how he used to play in school."

"Are there other sports you'd rather be playing?"

Ben looked up. "Well, a few of my friends are doing the running club that Mr. Caulfield and Ms. Lamb have started." He paused. "I don't think running would give me headaches. It would probably make me feel better."

Ms. Ernst knew that if Ben were truly re-experiencing concussion symptoms that any rigorous physical activity would be prohibited. But she suspected that Ben might be using symptoms as a ticket out of the fall football season. At the same time, she knew that her experiences with concussion was managing the educational side of helping students with concussion symptoms safely return to school. She was not a doctor and didn't want to make assumptions about Ben's medical condition.

"Have you talked with your parents about this?" she asked.

"No," said Ben. "My dad is all excited about me playing football this year. He even talked about maybe helping coach my team."

Ms. Ernst talked a bit more with Ben and together they decided she would speak to his mother before the end of the school day to share Ben's reluctance about resuming play on the football team. His mother was, in fact, relieved, as she did not want Ben playing football anymore either.

"His dad got his chance to play when he was in high school," she said. "This is Ben's life and he gets a say in the sport he wants to play."

REFERENCES

Collins, M., Lovell, M. R., Iverson, G. L., Ide, T., & Maroon, J. (2006). Examining concussion rates and return to play in high school football players wearing newer helmet technology: A three year prospective cohort study. *Neurosurgery, 58*(2), 275–286. doi:10.1227/01.NEU.0000200441.92742.46.

Halstead, M. E., McAvoy, K., Devore, C. D., Carl, R., Lee, M., Logan, K., ... Council on School Health (2013). Returning to learning following a concussion. *Official Journal of the American Pediatrics, 132*(5), 948–957. doi:10.1542/Peds.2013-2867.

Heinz, W. (2012). Return to function: Academic accommodations after a sports-related concussion. *The OA Update, 4*(2), 16–18.

Individuals with Disabilities Education Improvement Act, 20 U.S.C. § 1400 (2004).

McAvoy, K. (2012). Returning to learning: Going back to school following a concussion. *NASP Communique, 40*(6), 1, 23–25.

McAvoy, K., & Eagan Brown, B. E. (2015). *Get schooled on concussion*. Retrieved from http://www.getschooledonconcussions.com/topic-log.html

Nationwide Children's Hospital. (2012). *A school administrator's guide to academic concussion management*. Retrieved from http://www.nationwide childrens.org/concussions-in-the-classroom

Popoli, D. M., Burns, T. G., Meehan, W. P. III., & Reisner, A. (2014). CHOA concussion consensus: Establishing a uniform policy for academic accommodations. *Clinical Pediatrics, 53*(3), 217–224. doi:10.1177/0009922813499070.

Sady, M. D., Vaughan, C. G., & Gioia, G. A. (2011). School and the concussed youth: Recommendations for concussion education and management. *Physical Medicine and Rehabilitation Clinics of North America, 22*(4), 701–719. doi:10.1016/j.pmr.2011.08.008.

Section 504 of the Rehabilitation Act of 1973, 34 C.F.R. Part 104.

Zirkel, P. A., & Eagan Brown, B. E. (2015). K-12 students with concussions: A legal perspective. *The Journal of School Nursing, 31*(2), 99–109. doi:10.1177/1059840514521465.

CHAPTER 7

Prevention and Training

This book would not be complete without a chapter devoted to school-based concussion prevention efforts. These may include initiatives such as safety measures, sessions to train student athletes to recognize signs of concussion in teammates, and strategies for disseminating concussion information to school staff, families, and community members.

Engaging in sports and recreational activities has innumerable benefits for youth and it is not reasonable to expect we could prevent all brain injuries. However, some basic safety guidelines can make a significant impact in preventing them.

SCHOOL-BASED CONCUSSION PREVENTION PROGRAMS

Safety Measures

School personnel can conduct regular *safety reviews of play areas*, including both playgrounds and sporting areas. This includes making sure there is a soft surface to cushion falls under playground equipment, that there are railings around bleachers, and that the playing fields are well maintained. The physical space of the school should also be evaluated: Are there crosswalks to ensure safety of students who walk to school? Are there signs that indicate when floors are wet to prevent falls?

It is also important to provide *adequate staffing* to monitor recess and sporting events. These individuals must be trained not only in concussion recognition and response, but also in strategies for diffusing fights, managing risk-taking behaviors, and summoning help when needed. Officials monitoring youth sports need to call penalties when players break the rules. Otherwise, players will believe they can aggressively go after other players, executing moves that can endanger their opponents.

Both in recreational activities and in sports, there should be *guidelines and enforcement of rules*. Techniques used in sports should be age appropriate. For example, body checking is prohibited in many primary-age youth sports organizations. In sports that do allow physical contact, players should be proactively instructed in safe body alignment and techniques. They should also be encouraged to increase their awareness of what is going on around them, which can help reduce unexpected body hits that can cause concussions.

Some youth sports organizations have a "hit count," which is a limit to the number of head contacts a player experiences over a given time period. While such a policy makes good intuitive sense, it is also an example of a safety measure that still needs more scientific study to clarify its validity as a policy or recommendation.

Physical education programs should include lessons that emphasize safety, including the need for safety equipment, the correct use of such equipment, and rules of play. A director of physical education should provide leadership in class instruction, competition, and activities that are part of the school physical education (PE) program and ensure that safety measures are followed during such classes.

There are also recommendations for safety measures that are not currently required in a number of youth sports. Such reforms recommended by Dr. Robert Cantu, author of the 2012 book *Concussion and Our Kids* include:

- No tackle football before age 14
- No body checking in youth hockey before age 14
- No heading in soccer until age 14
- For youth baseball, require chin straps and restrict head-first slides

The age of 14 is not necessarily a "magical" age, but it is used for a few reasons. By age 14, a child's neck is stronger and the body is better able to keep the head steady during a body slam. The brain is also more mature; the fatty myelin coating on the nerves in the brain more effectively protect it from damage. At the age of 14, youth are also better able to make decisions for themselves related to what sports they want to play and what risks they want to take.

Safety measures can also be put in place related to the amount of contact expected during practice drills, as many concussions are sustained not only in competitive games, but during practices and scrimmages.

Carly

In reviewing their playground safety measures, Carly's school administrators found some areas for improvement. While everyone agreed that free play time—including climbing on age-appropriate equipment—was important, they determined that a softer surface needed to be installed below the climbing equipment. There was also a need for better training opportunities for playground aides and office staff in concussion recognition and response.

Protective Gear

Student athletes of all ages need *adequate protective gear*, such as helmets and mouth guards. However, contrary to what some individuals may believe, there is no research supporting the use of mouth guards to prevent concussions. And while helmets can protect against more severe brain injuries and fractures, they do not prevent all concussions (see Concussion Myths and Misconceptions in Chapter 1).

In recent years, the use of soft headgear products in sports that do not require helmets, such as girls' soccer, has become popular. The National Federation of State High School Associations (NFHS) Sports Medicine Advisory Committee (CMAC) developed a position statement (2013) regarding these products to address misperceptions regarding their performance in preventing concussions.

The statement indicates that soft or padded headgear products are not considered effective equipment for preventing concussions. Wearing such headgear is not scientifically or medically supported, thus it should not be considered as a valid way to decrease concussion incidence or expedite the return to play process. Further, wearing soft or padded headgear in non-helmeted sports may provide a false sense of security in athletes, parents, and coaches, thereby minimizing their focus on the importance of avoiding head impact and reporting concussion symptoms.

It is important that *athletic gear be appropriately fitted*. This includes ensuring that footwear fits appropriately and is the right type for the activity at hand. Young children who cannot tie their shoes well should have Velcro closures or have an adult double-knot their laces.

Because helmets can offer some protection against certain types of concussive blows, their addition can be helpful in sports that do not currently require helmets, such as field hockey and girls' lacrosse (Cantu & Hyman, 2012). Many girls participating in these sports sustain facial injuries, skull fractures, and other types of brain injuries. While some leagues have safety rules, such as no sticks above the knees, violations of this rule happen in most games and can, of course, result in concussions and other injuries to the head and face.

Athletic Programs

School districts' athletic programs can implement a number of safety measures to help make school sports safer for all participants. Preseason/beginning-of-year baseline testing, such as ImPACT, can provide preinjury measurement of cognitive abilities (see Chapter 4 for a discussion on this and other computerized neurocognitive tests) and help coaches, athletic trainers, medical personnel, and parents determine when a child is ready to safely return to athletic play.

Coaches can also be better trained in exercises that help strengthen their athletes; they can also conduct drills to enhance players' awareness of what is going on around them. Girls' coaches can explore the benefits of neck strengthening exercises for female athletes and better understand the type of exercises that can achieve this goal.

Further, a recent study indicated that only 70% of responding public high schools provided athletic trainers at sports competitions and practices and only 37% of public high schools had a full-time athletic trainer (Pryor et al., 2015). Not all high school associations require that a trainer be present at athletic competitions. This is often due to the high cost.

Changing the Culture

Increasing rates of concussion reporting will be an uphill battle as long as athletes continue to be immersed in a culture that praises "playing through the pain." It is crucial that players themselves be taught both how to prevent injuries as well as how to recognize and respond to known and suspected concussions. Student athletes need to see the signs not only in themselves, but also in their teammates.

A person with a brain injury is notorious for lacking judgment—it's one of the defining features—but a teammate who saw a concussive blow that a coach may have missed, or who heard the student complaining of dizziness in the locker room, can be tremendously helpful in getting that injured teammate the necessary medical care.

Unfortunately, many athletes would rather have their injured teammate play through a game if it means the difference between a win and a loss. School professionals can help change the concussion culture by encouraging the reporting of known and suspected concussions to responsible adults who can then connect with the concussion team leader.

Students need to learn self-advocacy as well. The term *health literacy* applies to one's understanding of one's own health condition or injury in order to make appropriate health decisions (Manganello, 2008). If students better understand their injuries, including how symptoms can affect their academic performance, emotional well-being, and physical condition, they might better advocate for their own needs. Thus, children and adolescents should be educated on the importance of disclosing a head injury and following concussion-management recommendations.

TRAINING GUIDELINES

In addition to safety measures, education can help reduce concussions. Even when concussion management procedures and return-to-play guidelines are in place, many high schools do not provide frequent concussion education to their athletes. Without concussion education regarding how students' injuries may affect their daily activities, athletes and nonathletes alike often return to the academic demands of school prematurely.

Schools—particularly middle and high schools—should require coaches of youth athletic activities to complete a concussion recognition education course each year. Such training should also be required of volunteer coaches at club and recreation facilities, as well as athletic leagues that sponsor youth sports. This training can include information on signs and symptoms of concussion, how to obtain medical attention in the event of a suspected concussion, risk factors of untreated concussions, and how to properly return an athlete who has sustained a concussion to athletic activity.

It is also important to keep in mind that many students' concussions were not sustained in athletic activities. Therefore, training is recommended for all school staff who supervise play and recreation. This includes teachers (particularly physical education teachers), aides, office staff, related service personnel, administrators, and nursing staff. Such training should include information on both recognizing and responding to known and suspected concussions, guidelines for participating in a school-based concussion team, and ways to make adjustments to the school environment to meet students' needs upon return to school.

Leaders of such trainings can provide resources such as this book or they can turn to reputable online training sources, such as the Centers for Disease Control and Prevention (www.cdc.gov/concussion) or the Brain101 "Concussion Playbook" (http://brain101.orcasinc.com), which has videos and resources for coaches, educators, parents, and students. Those conducting school-based trainings might construct a child-based concussion scenario based on their work or personal experience and walk participants through appropriate response steps. They can also have participants engage in small group role plays. In these groups, each participant would assume specific roles (e.g., student, teacher, parent, school psychologist, nurse, administrator, coach) and act out a concussion response scenario, such as determining appropriate adjustments to the school environment upon the child's return after sustaining a concussion.

Damien

> Damien's school had no concussion team when he returned to school after his car accident. The problems he encountered inspired his school principal to implement a concussion team model and return-to-learn strategies in his building. The principal orchestrated the design and implementation of a policy that was later adopted by the school board. This included a concussion team training for the district administrators, school nurses, school psychologists, school counselors, and athletic trainer.

Following are several reputable concussion training resources that are available online:

1. **Brain101** (http://brain101.orcasinc.com):

    This site is a user friendly, visually appealing, and straightforward resource to guide the planning, training, and implementation of a school-wide concussion management system and team. The site includes resources specific to coaches, educators, parents, and teen athletes. The site includes brief informative/training videos, which are accompanied by questions regarding how to handle concussion-related management in the school. The site also includes practical resources to assist in implementing a concussion management plan schoolwide, including a signs and symptoms of concussion handout, staff notification letter, return-to-activities guide, concussion management team's roles and responsibilities, and more.

2. **BrainSTEPS** (www.brainsteps.net; Brain Injury Association of Pennsylvania, Inc., the Pennsylvania Department of Education, & the Pennsylvania Department of Health, 2007):

    BrainSTEPS is a brain injury school re-entry consulting program; STEPS stands for Strategies Teaching Educators, Parents, and Students. Although this is a Pennsylvania-based program, many of the resources on the site can be applied anywhere. Further, it is an outstanding example of positive collaboration—in this case among the Department of Health, Department of Education, and Brain Injury Association—for addressing issues associated with youth concussions. This site includes information on concussion signs and symptoms, concussion teams in schools, and the implementation of return to school procedures.

    BrainSTEPS.net offers a variety of webinars, including Concussions in the Classroom—Return to Learning, IEPs and Effective Program Planning for Students with Traumatic Brain Injury, Intervention for Adolescents With Acquired Brain Injury, and Strategies for Executive Skills Development in Students With TBI. The webinars are accompanied by classroom resources for teachers and concussion team members.

3. **Centers for Disease Control and Prevention—Heads Up to Schools** (www.cdc.gov/headsup/schools/index.html; CDC, 2015):

    This site provides resources on concussion signs and symptoms, promoting awareness, and tips for parents on how to provide care to students who have sustained concussion. The CDC provides fact sheets about concussion that are directed toward parents, school professionals, and coaches, most of which are downloadable in both English and Spanish. The site also provides information about how to return students to the classroom after sustaining a concussion, and provides PDFs with tips for teachers to assist in returning students to the classroom.

The Heads Up program also includes concussion awareness flyers that can be customized, downloaded, and posted in schools. These flyers are simple, visually appealing, and include information about common symptoms and the importance of reporting concussion symptoms to a school professional.

Detailed information regarding helmet safety can also be found on the CDC's Heads Up to Schools site. Fact sheets on appropriate helmet fit, usage, and coverage are available for many different types of sports (helmets for skateboarding, ice hockey, football, bike riding, etc.). Three brief online concussion training courses are also available on this site; one for clinicians, one for youth sports coaches, and one for high school sports coaches.

4. **The Center on Brain Injury Research and Training** (http://cbirt.org; University of Oregon, n.d.):

   The Center on Brain Injury Research and Training provides a number of presentations on brain injury research, many of which involve how to support students who have sustained a traumatic brain injury, how to involve parents in concussion care, and research-based interventions for students who have sustained concussions. The site also includes resources for families, educators, and service providers based on best practice recommendations for working with students with concussion.

5. **Colorado Kids Brain Injury Resource Network** (http://cokidswithbraininjury.com; Brain Injury Networking Team, 2015):

   Cokidswithbraininjury.com provides information geared toward educators and professionals, as well as information for parents on how to support students who have sustained concussion. The site includes detailed yet simple resources and tools that can simply be printed and used in schools; examples include: Brain Check Survey, Comprehensive Health Assessment, and Brain Injury Observation Form. The site also includes helpful resources such as "Key Terms" for concussion in schools. Much of this site is specific to Colorado-based resources and law, however, the site also includes national law updates and national resources such as the CDC, and Brain Injury Association of America.

6. **Get Schooled on Concussions** (www.getschooledonconcussions.com; McAvoy & Eagan Brown, 2015):

   Get Schooled on Concussions is a website that focuses on "return-to-learn" recommendations, "written *by* educators *for* educators." The main objective of this site is to provide teachers, administrators, school nurses, school mental health counselors, and parents with one-page fact sheets on concussion recovery in the classroom. This site provides educators and school professionals with to-the-point fact sheets on important aspects of, returning to academics such as: What to Do About Work Output, When to Write a Section 504 Plan, What to Do About Tests, and Academic and Symptom Monitoring. This site also provides archived return-to-learn trainings, as well as information on upcoming trainings.

7. **Nationwide Children's Hospital Concussion Clinic** (www.nationwidechildrens.org/concussions; Nationwide Children's Hospital, n.d.):

   Nationwide Children's Hospital provides medical and management services for children and their families who have sustained many kinds of illnesses, injuries, or disabilities. This site directs the reader to their concussion clinic and concussion resources page. This site provides resources on a variety of topics including, but not limited to, easy-to-use tools for parents, coaches, educators, school administrators, and athletes; a guide to the concussion management team (including roles, responsibilities, etc.); information regarding baseline neurocognitive testing; current articles on concussion; and so on. The site also includes a page on frequently asked questions regarding Ohio's concussion law.

8. **University Interscholastic League/National Federation of State High School Associations—Concussion Oversight Team** (www.uiltexas.org/health/concussions; University Interscholastic League, n.d.):

   This site provides information regarding the suggested acknowledgment, supervision, and management/treatment of concussion in schools, as suggested by the National Federation of State High School Associations (NFHS) and Texas law. The site also includes a link to a free course titled Concussion in Sports—What You Need to Know, which is supported by NFHS and CDC, that focuses on providing resources to help educate coaches, officials, parents, and students on concussion awareness, recognition, and proper management. Though many of the resources on this site are specific to the law and protocol of Texas schools, the site includes return-to-play resources, a concussion management protocol, and suggested guidelines for concussion management that can be applicable to any school system.

PARENTS

This book has described how parents are key members of the school-based concussion team. They know their child better than anyone and they can notice small behavioral changes more readily than others might, particularly a physician who may only see the child for annual well-child visits. Parents might notice changes in sleeping and eating, reactions to minor stressors, and overall demeanor. Therefore, school personnel should always ask parents, "What have you noticed?" when monitoring a student's progress through concussion recovery.

While parents should not be expected to diagnose concussions, they do need to know when to take their child to a doctor for evaluation for a suspected concussion. The sooner a child receives proper treatment, the better the likelihood for a positive outcome. Therefore, it is crucial that parents be involved in district-level training and prevention initiatives.

Parents can be taught some of the simple assessment techniques that were described in Chapter 4. They can ask simple questions to check their child's short-term memory, such as "What was the score of the game?" "What school were you playing against?" and "What do you remember about what happened?"

It is important that parents realize that many doctors have not received adequate training in diagnosing concussions. One colleague's local hospital is notorious for sending students home from the emergency department declaring that because the child's CT scan was clear, they didn't have a concussion (see Chapter 1 myths). Because concussion training is relatively new to the medical field, most doctors currently in practice received little or no education about it during their training. Instead, they are receiving information about concussion through professional readings and continuing education seminars (if at all). Thus, it's important that when selecting a doctor, parents not only consider the doctor they have used for years, but that they ask about the doctor's training in concussions. In many cases, parents are well advised to seek out a concussion specialist to care for their child.

Parents will usually be their child's strongest advocates, eager to find out what their son or daughter needs and how they can facilitate the recovery process. However, in some situations, parents may not understand the serious repercussions that can come with too much activity while a concussion is still healing. If their child is an athlete, parents may want them to get back into the game, to hold onto their status as the star on the soccer team, or to maintain their trajectory toward a football scholarship. This can be a difficult dynamic for school staff members to navigate. In all cases, it can be helpful to have the release of information (ROI) signed to allow conversation between a physician and the concussion team leader. In this type of case, the physician—as long as he or she is well educated about concussions and the recovery process—can often give additional support and guidance.

Parents can be a tremendous help to their children throughout the recovery process, as well as in terms of helping prevent concussions in the first place. Again, most parents are active partners in the recovery process. However, if the student and/or the family are noncompliant members of the concussion team and refuse to follow recommendations, it is important that the CTL documents situations and correspondence. The CTL should also document the school's efforts. Having clear communication and a supportive relationship can help ensure compliance.

Ben

When Ben sustained his concussion playing football, his father was upset that he was not allowed to resume practice and play. The following year, Ben's father continued to present some difficulties to the school team.

"This is ridiculous," Mr. Davidson grumbled. "I played football for 10 years and got my share of dings, but I turned out fine."

"You have trouble remembering things from time to time," Mrs. Davidson murmured.

"Who doesn't!" Mr. Davidson snapped. "The truth is, the boy just needs to toughen up—and football is the way he's gonna do it!"

"It sounds like football was a really important part of your life when you were in school," the school psychologist said. "I was the same way with ice hockey. What is it about football that you like the most for Ben?"

"I want him to be part of a team," Mr. Davidson said evenly, "To work hard, to compete, and to be a man."

"Ben doesn't seem as enthusiastic about football, but he is very excited about the possibility of joining the running club instead," added his school counselor, Ms. Ernst. "He'd get a lot of things out of it that you're looking for in football—teamwork, competition, strength development—and it would be good conditioning for football or another sport he chooses down the road."

NEXT STEPS

Some readers of this book may be learning much of this information for the first time. Others may be reading it as part of a required course or for professional development with a school team. Given that readers are coming at this text from a variety of angles, keep in mind the following general recommendations for next steps:

- **Establish a concussion team at your school:** Review the key personnel recommended for participation in a concussion team in Chapter 3. Talk with your school or district administration to gain support for implementation of a team model.
- **Designate a CTL:** A school-based concussion team is only as strong as its leader. The professional who serves in this role will vary from school to school. *Maybe this person is you.* Regardless, keep in mind that if the designated CTL changes jobs or moves to a different school, a new person needs to be appointed and existing cases (including those being followed from previous years) need to be transitioned.
- **Educate your community:** Help provide information to all students, parents, athletic staff, and educators about how concussions can affect learning, behavior, and health. An online resource for this is *Brain 101: The Concussion Playbook* (http://brain101.orcasinc.com), which teaches students what to look for and encourages them to tell an adult if they think they have a concussion. There is an excellent 15-minute video on this site—encourage sharing of this video with students.
- **Define your concussion protocol:** Ensure that there is a written protocol or manual for your school and that all concussion team members understand their responsibilities.

A FINAL NOTE

Physical rest and cognitive rest are both essential for concussion recovery. With appropriate response and treatment, more than 80% of students with concussions recover within 3 weeks (Collins, Lovell, Iverson, Ide, & Maroon, 2006). However, if concussive injuries are not managed appropriately, recovery time can be prolonged and academic difficulties can persist. Thus, it is essential to have a school-based concussion management plan in place while a child heals. Such a plan includes appropriate environmental and academic adjustments, a mechanism for progress monitoring, and communication among school personnel, medical personnel, and families.

As much as some of us would like to, we cannot wrap kids in bubble wrap to send them out into the world. Engaging in physical play, playing sports, and learning to drive a car are all ways youth can sustain concussions, but they're also important parts of both child development and our culture. Climbing on monkey bars can help develop a child's coordination, playing on the baseball team can help develop sportsmanship, and driving a car can help develop a sense of independence. At the same time, with any of these activities comes risk of injury, and with injury comes the responsibility for an appropriate, coordinated response.

NEW PATHS

Some concussions can derail a student athlete's projected path. This book concludes with Julia's story, and the new path that she forged in the aftermath of her postconcussion syndrome.

Julia

Julia had always been a high-achieving student academically as well as athletically, but after her last concussion, her grades began to slip. Julia had a complex constellation of symptoms, including headaches, fatigue, poor memory, nervousness, and irritability. With help from her school-based concussion team, her teachers, and her parents, Julia received appropriate adjustments at school that facilitated her recovery.

Julia had dreams of a soccer scholarship to a big state university. However, after her last concussion, it was apparent that an athletic career was not in her future. Julia felt lost and angry and confused. Not only had her academic performance suffered as a result of her concussion, but she lost much of her sense of belonging and social circle, which had all centered on her soccer and basketball team.

"Sometimes I feel like I've moved to a new school," she told her mother. "I feel like I have to make friends all over again."

"Your friends still care about you so much," said her mother, who proceeded to name specific friends and the things they had done to stay connected to Julia during her recovery.

"I know," Julia sighed, "but it's just not the same. I mean, when I'm around them, and they're talking about something that happened at practice or on the bus on the way to a game, I feel so left out. It's like they have these inside jokes that I'll never be part of again."

Julia's mother encouraged her to stay connected to her old friends and teammates, but also to explore new social groups and areas of interest.

"It's a great opportunity," she said, "to learn how to do something new... something you've always wanted to do but haven't had time for."

Julia's summers had always been dominated by sports camps and conditioning. During the summer after her junior year, she and her mother took a 2-week trip to California and spent a great deal of time reading and relaxing at their local swimming pool.

"It was this great opportunity to spend time together before Julia's senior year, and before she launches into the rest of her life," Julia's mother told the Mrs. Beck, the school counselor. "And she's started taking guitar lessons—she seems to have a real gift for it."

"That's very positive," nodded Mrs. Beck.

"I'm not saying everything is rosy and perfect," said Julia's mom. "She still seems down from time to time, but her schoolwork has improved and she's looking at more colleges over the break. She can see opportunities there, too—although she'll need more student loans without the possibility of a scholarship, but she's not just limited to schools with strong soccer programs anymore."

Julia continued to pursue her love of guitar during the rest of high school and even recorded some songs that received thousands of hits on YouTube. She remained close with several of her former teammates and also made new friends who were involved with her school's music program, including her new boyfriend, Danny. When a freshman at her school sustained a similar injury and was sidelined from play for the rest of the soccer season, Mrs. Beck connected the two young ladies over lunch so Julia could share her story—and her strategies—with someone else.

REFERENCES

Brain Injury Association of Pennsylvania Inc., the Pennsylvania Department of Education, & the Pennsylvania Department of Health. (2007). BrainSTEPS. Retrieved from http://www.brainsteps.net

Brain Injury Networking Team. (2015). Colorado kids brain injury resource network. Retrieved from http://cokidswithbraininjury.com

Cantu, R., & Hyman, M. (2012). *Concussion and our kids: America's leading expert on how to protect young athletes and keep sports safe.* New York, NY: Houghton Mifflin Harcourt Publishing Company.

Centers for Disease Control and Prevention. (2015). Center for disease control and prevention: CDC 24/7: Saving lives, protecting people. Retrieved from http://www.cdc.gov/headsup/index.html

Collins, M., Lovell, M. R., Iverson, G. L., Ide, T., & Maroon, J. (2006). Examining concussion rates and return to play in high school football players wearing newer helmet technology: A three year prospective cohort study. *Neurosurgery, 58*(2), 275–286. doi:10.1227/01.NEU.0000200441.92742.46

Manganello, J. A. (2008). Health literacy and adolescents: A framework and agenda for future research. *Health Education Research, 23*(5), 840–847. doi:10.1093/her/cym069

McAvoy, K., & Eagan Brown, B. (2015). Get schooled on concussions: Return to learn (RTL). Retrieved from http://www.getschooledonconcussions.com

National Federation of State High School Associations Sports Medicine Advisory Committee (2013). *Soft or padded headgear in non-helmeted sports position statement.* Retrieved from https://www.nfhs.org/media/1015199/2013-nfhs-smac-postion-statement-on-soft-headgear-1.pdf

Nationwide Children's Hospital. (n.d.). Nationwide children's: When your child needs a hospital, everything matters. Retrieved from http://www.nationwidechildrens.org/concussions

Pryor, R. R., Casa, D. J., Vandermark, L. W., Stearns, R. L., Attanasio, S. M., Fontaine, G. J., & Wafer, A. M. (2015). Athletic training services in public secondary schools: A benchmark study. *Journal of Athletic Training, 50*(2), 156–162. doi:10.4085/1062-5060-50.2.03

University Interscholastic League. (n.d.). Health and safety: Concussions and concussion management protocol requirements and information. Retrieved from http://www.uiltexas.org/health/concussions

University of Oregon. (n.d.). The center on brain injury research & training. Retrieved from http://cbirt.org

INDEX

Academic Adjustment Plan, 54
academic adjustments, 119–120, 123–126
academic team members, 45–47
ACE. *See* Acute Concussion Evaluation
Acute Concussion Evaluation (ACE), 72–73
   care plan, 113–114
   instructions, 73
adjustments, postconcussion, 115–118
   cognitive symptoms, for students with, 118–126
administrator, on concussion team, 46
adolescence, as risk factor, 9
Alzheimer's disease, 35
American Academy of Neurology's Concussion Quick Check, Version 2.2.0, 78
assessment
   clinical evaluation, 79–80
   future of, newer techniques, 91–92
   neurocognitive computerized testing, 74–75
   ongoing, at school, 80–91
   sideline assessment, 75–77
   smartphone and tablet apps, 77–79
athletes, and concussion, 106–107
Athletic Director (AD), on concussion team, 50
athletic programs, safety measures, 140
athletic trainer (AT), on concussion team, 48

Balance Error Scoring System (BESS), 76
BESS. *See* Balance Error Scoring System
Brain101, 142–143

brain injuries, 22, 36–37.
   See also mild traumatic brain injury; traumatic brain injury
BrainSTEPS, 143

case management, 80
case manager. *See* concussion team leader
CDC. *See* Centers for Disease Control and Prevention
Center on Brain Injury Research and Training, 144
Centers for Disease Control and Prevention (CDC), 143
   Acute Concussion Evaluation (ACE), 72–73
   concussion signs and symptoms checklist, 67–71
   estimation of concussions, 4
   "Heads Up" App, Version 1.0, 77
   Heads Up to Schools, 143–144
childhood, as risk factor for concussions, 8–9
Child SCAT3, 76
child vomiting, as sign of concussion, 12
chronic traumatic encephalopathy (CTE), 9, 34–36
   suicide and, 36–37
   medial temporal lobe, effects on, 35
clinical evaluation, of concussion, 79
coach, on concussion team, 49
cognitive exertion, 121
   process of, 101
cognitive rest, in recovery, 97–98
cognitive symptoms, adjustments for students with, 118–122
cognitive therapy, 100
college student, effects of concussion, 29–30

INDEX

Colorado Kids Brain Injury Resource Network, 144
communication, concussion team, 135
computerized neurocognitive tests, 44–45, 49, 66, 106
concussion team, 41–42
  model, 40
    management process, 52–58
    parents, working with, 59–60
    school community, educating, 58–59
    student privacy, 61–63
    sustainability of, 64
  structures
    academic team members, 45–46
    athletic team members, 49–50
    family, 43–44
    medical team members, 47–48
    with one versus two leaders, 52
concussion team leader (CTL), 40, 50–51, 148
  case tracking, 81
Consensus Statement on Concussion in Sport, 106
CTE. *See* chronic traumatic encephalopathy
CTL. *See* concussion team leader
cumulative trauma, increased risk of, 9

danger signs, 26–27
decision making, in return to academics, 126–127
Dynamic Vision Test, 78

elementary school student, effects of concussions, 27–28
extracurricular involvement, in recovery period, 127

family, and concussion team, 43–44
Family Educational Rights and Privacy Act (FERPA), 40, 62–63
FERPA. *See* Family Educational Rights and Privacy Act
football, and concussions, 2, 6, 7, 9, 15

Get Schooled on Concussions, 144–145
grade levels, effects of concussions
  college student, 29–30
  elementary school student, 27–28
  high school student, 29
  middle school student, 28

Health Insurance Portability and Accountability Act (HIPPA), 61
health literacy, 141
helmets, to prevent concussions, 12–13, 77, 139–140
high school student, effects of concussions, 29
HIPPA. *See* Health Insurance Portability and Accountability Act

IDEA. *See* Individuals with Disabilities Education Improvement Act
IEP. *See* individualized education program
Immediate Post-Concussion Assessment and Cognitive Testing (ImPACT), 74, 75, 78, 140
ImPACT. *See* Immediate Post-Concussion Assessment and Cognitive Testing
individualized education program (IEP), 115, 131, 134
Individuals with Disabilities Education Improvement Act (IDEA), 62, 131
informal interviews, for concussion symptoms, 83–89

K-D Test. *See* King-Devick Test
King-Devick Test (K-D Test), 77
   Version 1.0, 78

legislation and policies, 16–17
loss of consciousness and, 12

management process,
   concussion, 52–58
medial temporal lobe, affecting, 35
medical members, concussion
   team, 47–48
mental exertion, 117
middle school student, effects of
   concussions, 28
mild traumatic brain injury
   (mTBI), 1, 4, 73
misconceptions, about
   concussions, 11–16
modifications, to school
   environment, 115
mTBI. *See* mild traumatic brain
   injury
MTSS. *See* multitiered system of
   support
multiple concussions, 30–31
multiple injuries, risk of, 31
multitiered system of support
   (MTSS), 131
myths, about concussions, 11–16

National Federation of State
   High School Associations
   (NFHS), 145
   Injury Surveillance System, 5
National Federation of State High
   School Associations—
   Concussion Oversight
   Team, 145
National Football League (NFL), 34
Nationwide Children's Hospital
   Concussion Clinic, 145
neurocognitive computerized
   testing, for concussion, 74–75
   drawbacks, 74

neurological changes, 21–23
neuronal connection, effects on, 22
NFHS. *See* National Federation
   of State High School
   Associations
NFL. *See* National Football League
noise avoidance, postconcussion,
   117–118
nonmedication treatments, 100
nonsports concussions
   cause of, 7
   rates of, 5

observations, of concussion
   symptoms, 89–90
OHI. *See* other health impairment
ongoing concussion assessment at
   schools
   case management, 80
   informal interviews for
     symptoms, 83–89
   observations, and assessment of
     recovery, 89–90
other health impairment (OHI), 134
overstimulating environments,
   avoidance, 117–118
   symptom progress
     monitoring, 81–83
over-the-counter medications,
   99–100

parents
   and guardians as concussion team
     members, 43–44
   role in assessment and recovery,
     146–147
PAR's Concussion Recognition and
   Response, 77
pathophysiological changes, 21–23
PCS. *See* postconcussion syndrome
peer relations, monitoring, 123
persistent and severe difficulties
   brain injury, 36–37
   chronic traumatic
     encephalopathy, 34–36